Surgery of the Small Bowel

Kirby I. Bland • Michael G. Sarr
Markus W. Büchler • Attila Csendes
Oliver James Garden • John Wong
(Editors)

Surgery of the Small Bowel

Handbooks in General Surgery

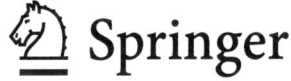 Springer

Editors

Kirby I. Bland
University of Alabama
Birmingham
Department of Surgery
Birmingham Alabama
USA

Michael G. Sarr
Mayo Clinic
Division of Gastroenterologic &
General Surgery
Rochester Minnesota
USA

Markus W. Büchler
Universitätsklinikum Heidelberg
Chirurgische Klinik
Abt. Allgemeine, Viszerale und
Unfallchirurgie
Heidelberg
Germany

Attila Csendes
University of Chile
Clinical Hospital
Department of Surgery
Santiago
Chile

Oliver James Garden
University of Edinburgh
Royal Infirmary
Department of Surgery
Edinburgh
United Kingdom

John Wong
Queen Mary Hospital
Department of Surgery
Hong Kong

ISBN 978-1-84996-371-8   e-ISBN 978-1-84996-372-5
DOI 10.1007/978-1-84996-372-5
Springer London Dordrecht Heidelberg New York

British Library Cataloguing in Publication Data
A catalogue record for this book is available from the British Library

Library of Congress Control Number: 2010937964

Cover design: eStudioCalamar Figueres/Berlin

Printed on acid-free paper

Springer is part of Springer Science+Business Media (www.springer.com)

Preface

The editors designed the original textbook, *General Surgery: Principles and International Practice,* from which this shorter paperback monograph on surgery of the small bowel was taken to be an accessible, concise, and state-of-the-art volume that explores and documents evolutionary principles in the practice of surgery. This work is aimed at the general surgeon and the resident in training. The scientific community continues to witness extraordinary advances in the therapy of both benign and malignant surgical diseases of various organ sites. Much of this progress has been evident over the past decade with new concepts and techniques of management that allow the surgeon to integrate this discipline with medicine, pharmacology, immunology, biostatistics, pathology, genetics, medical and radiation oncology, and diagnostic radiology and imaging. Further, each of these major disciplines contributes a small component for the diagnostic and therapeutic approaches to clinical care; hence the comprehensive planning, integration, and provision of patient care throughout the preoperative, intraoperative, and postoperative phases of care remains essential in the successful practice of our specialty.

The editors acknowledge that the aim of this work is to provide an illustrative, instructive, and comprehensive review that depicts the rationale of basic operative principles essential to surgical therapy. In organizing this monograph, the editors chose authors renowned in the disciplines for illustrating, forming, and depicting in a comprehensive fashion the surgical therapy expectant for metabolic, infectious, endocrine, and neoplastic abnormalities in adult and pediatric patients **from a truly international and multi-continental**

perspective. The editors and authors were chosen carefully from across geographies and also from multi-cultural and diverse locations. While the authors consider this text to be inclusive regarding the technical and operative conditions for perioperative care in this field, its purpose should not be intended to replace standard textbooks of surgery nor should it be considered complete in its coverage of pathophysiologic disorders. In contrast, this monograph is organized to familiarize practicing surgeons, residents, and fellows with state-of-the-art surgical principles and techniques essential to contemporary practice. Therefore, the tenor of this monograph on surgery of the small bowel has been developed to coexist with other major surgical reference texts that are dedicated—some in more comprehensive fashion—to the therapy of individual organs of systemic diseases. This monograph is much more a "working text" for the practicing surgeon with emphasis on diagnosis and treatment of small bowel disorders. Along with this monograph, nine other paperback monographs are available and focus on the general principles of surgery, trauma, critical care, esophagus and stomach, colorectal, liver and biliary, pancreas and spleen, oncology, and endocrine organs, all adapted from the primary textbook—*General Surgery: Principles and International Practice.*

The chapters in this monograph on surgery of the small bowel include a condensed bibliography of highly selective journal articles, reviews, and text. In this manner of attempting to be concise, we hope to provide a precise focus for the education of the reader relative to accepted surgical principles involved in patient care. Moreover, the editors have sought to provide a counterpoint view for the selection of therapy by presenting at the opening of each chapter a list of "Pearls and Pitfalls" that highlight particular concerns or controversies. The chapters provide pertinent, though not exhaustive, summaries of anatomy and physiology, a history of surgical illness, and stages of operative approaches with relevant technical considerations outlined in an easily understandable manner. Complications are reviewed when appropriate for the organ system, diseases, and problem. The text is supported amply by line drawings and photographs that depict anatomic or technical principles. The editors have made every attempt to minimize duplicative or repetitive discussions except when controversial or state-of-the-art issues are presented. Moreover, the editors have attempted to ensure that accurate presentations and illustrations depict properly the most complex problems confronted by the general surgeon.

Finally, in an attempt to address advances in contemporary concepts, the text has been organized to address in detail expeditious, safe, and anatomically accurate operations and incorporate standard as well as evolving surgical principles and techniques. These principles have been tested in the clinics of valid scientific knowledge and are well supported by the time-tested approaches that have been provided by practicing surgeons. The editors are excited to be able to respond to the challenge of developing a truly international text and are indeed hopeful that our readers will find this focused monograph on surgery of the small bowel to be a repository of insight, useful, and timely information.

Kirby I. Bland
Michael G. Sarr
Markus W. Büchler
Attila Csendes
O. James Garden
John Wong

Contents

Contributors

Supreeta Arya, MD
Associate Professor and Consultant Radiologist,
Department of Radiodiagnosis, Tata Memorial Hospital,
Mumbai, India

Wing-Yan Au, MD, FRCPE
Professor, Department of Medicine, Queen Mary Hospital,
Hong Kong, China

Orlin N. Belyaev, MD
Assistant Physician, Department of Surgery,
St. Josef Hospital, Ruhr University, Bochum,
Bochum, Germany

Kathleen K. Christians, MD
Associate Professor of Surgery, Department of Surgery,
Medical College of Wisconsin, Milwaukee, WI, USA

Matthew R. Dixon, MD
Fellow, Department of Colon and Rectal Surgery,
University of Minnesota, St. Paul, MN, USA

David R. Farley, MD
Professor, Department of Surgery, Mayo Clinic Foundation,
Rochester, MN, USA

Victor W. Fazio, MB, MS, FRACS, FACS, FRCS
Rupert B, Turnbull Jr. MD Professor, Chairman,
Department of Colorectal Surgery, Cleveland Clinic
Foundation, Cleveland, OH, USA

Joaquim Gama-Rodrigues, MD, PhD
Associate Professor of Surgery,
Department of Gastroenterology, University of São Paulo,
São Paulo, Brazil

Jason F. Hall, MD
Department of Surgery, Harvard Medical School,
Massachusetts General Hospital, Boston, MA, USA

Richard Hodin, MD
Professor, Department of Surgery, Harvard Medical School,
Massachusetts General Hospital, Boston, MA, USA

Carlos Eduardo Jacob, MD, PhD
Department of Gastroenterology Digestive Surgery Unit
University of São Paulo Medical School São Paulo, Brazil

**Raymond H. S. Liang, MD, FRCPE, FRCPG, FRCP,
FRACP, FHKCP, FHKAM** (medicine)
S.H.Ho Professor in Haematology and Oncology,
Li Ka Shing Faculty of Medicine, University of Hong Kong,
Hong Kong, China

Sherry J. Lim, MD
Fellow, Surgical Oncology, University of Texas M D
Anderson Cancer Center, Houston, TX, USA

Reginald V. N. Lord, MD
Consultant Surgeon, Department of Surgery,
St. Vincent's Hospital, Sydney University of New South
Wales, Sydney, Australia

Christophe A. Müller, MD
Department of Surgery, St. Josef Hospital,
|Bochum Ruhr University, Bochum, Bochum, Germany

Elisabeth C. McLemore, MD
General Surgery Resident, Department of Colorectal
Surgery, Cleveland Clinic Florida, Weston, FL, USA

Mary F. Otterson, MD MS FACS
Professor of Surgery, Division of General Surgery,
Medical College of Wisconsin, Milwaukee, WI, USA

Peter W. T. Pisters, MD
Professor of Surgery, Department of Surgical Oncology,
University of Texas M D Anderson Cancer Center,
Houston, TX, USA

Igor Proscurshim, BS
Department of Gastroenterology, University of São Paulo
Medical School, São Paulo, Brazil

John R. Porterfield Jr., MD, MSPH
General Surgery Resident Department of Surgery Mayo
Clinic College of Medicine Rochester, MN, USA

Feza H. Remzi, MD, FACS, FASCRS
Department of Colorectal Surgery, Cleveland Clinic,
Cleveland, OH, USA

Götz M. Richter, MD
Professor, Department of Radiology, University of
Heidelberg, Heidelberg, Germany

Shailesh V. Shrikhande, MD, MBBS, MS
Associate Professor and Consultant Surgeon, Department
of Gastrointestinal Surgical Oncology, Tata Memorial
Hospital, Maharashtra, India

Lelan F. Sillin III, MD, MS (Ed), FACS
Professor of Surgery and Vice Chair of Educational Affairs,
Department of Surgery School of Medicine and Dentistry,
University of Rochester, Rochester, NY, USA

Michael J. Stamos, MD, FACS, FASCRS
Professor of Surgery, Chief, Division of Colon and Rectal
Surgery, Department of Surgery, UC Irvine Medical Center,
Orange, CA, USA

Jon S. Thompson, MD
Professor and Vice Chair, Department of Surgery,
University of Nebraska Medical Center, Omaha, NE, USA

Waldemar H. Uhl, MD, FRCS
Professor, Department of Surgery, St. Josef Hospital,
Bochum, Bochum, Germany

Jens Werner, MD
Professor of Surgery, Department of General and Visceral
Surgery, University of Heidelberg, Heidelberg, Germany

Tonia M. Young-Fadok, MD, MS, FACS, FASCRS
Professor of Surgery, Chair, Division of Colon and Rectal
Surgery, Mayo Clinic, Phoenix, AZ, USA

Part I
Benign

1
Small Bowel Obstruction

Orlin N. Belyaev, Christophe Müller, and Waldemar H. Uhl

Pearls and Pitfalls

- For patients with acute, crampy, abdominal pain and obstipation, always consider the possibility of small bowel obstruction (SBO).
- A detailed history, thorough physical examination, and characteristic findings on a plain abdominal film are usually sufficient to establish the diagnosis.
- Postoperative adhesions are the most common cause of SBO, followed by hernias and neoplasms.
- SBO should be differentiated from non-mechanical intestinal paralysis (ileus), especially in the postoperative period.
- The management of patients with SBO is based on intravenous resuscitation, nasogastric decompression, and expeditious surgery when necessary. "The sun should never rise and set on a SBO."
- All patients with complete bowel obstruction should immediately undergo operative intervention unless extraordinary circumstances such as terminal illness are present.
- A midline laparotomy is used as a standard. The surgical procedure should manage the intestinal segment at the site of the obstruction, the distended proximal bowel, and the underlying cause of SBO.
- A resection is the best and safest choice when doubt about bowel viability exists.

K.I. Bland et al. (eds.), *Surgery of the Small Bowel*,
DOI: 10.1007/978-1-84996-372-5_1,
© Springer-Verlag London Limited 2011

- Postoperative, immediate bowel stimulation with proki- netics, early mobilization, and removal of the nasogastric tube accelerate patient's recovery.
- The best prophylaxis of postoperative adhesions includes gentle handling of the distended intestine, avoiding intro- duction of foreign materials, careful repair of serosal defects, and copious lavage of the peritoneal cavity. Efficacy of all other methods, such as resorbable barrier membranes or chemical agents, has not yet been proven by randomized controlled trials.
- Decreasing the incidence of SBO requires an intentional search for and early elective repair of all abdominal wall hernias.

Introduction

Definition and Etiology

Small bowel obstruction is an interruption of the normal flow of luminal contents at the level of the small bowel caused by a mechanical blockage. SBO is a common medical prob- lem and accounts for one of every five acute surgical admis- sions. The increasing number of patients undergoing laparotomy and their prolonged life expectancy have lead to peritoneal adhesions being the leading cause of SBO world- wide. Hernias and metastatic colorectal and ovarian cancer are the next most common causes. Adhesions, hernias, and metastatic cancer account for about 90% of all cases of SBO (Table 1.1).

SBO can be incomplete (partial) or complete and simple or strangulated. A simple SBO is present when the bowel is occluded at a single point leading to proximal intestinal dilata- tion and distal intestinal decompression. Vascular compromise is unlikely with simple SBO. A closed-loop SBO is present when a bowel segment is occluded at two points, so that both the proximal and distal loops, as well as the bowel's mesentery are entrapped by a single constrictive lesion. A strangulated SBO is observed when the blood supply to a closed-loop

TABLE 1.1. Causes of mechanical small bowel obstruction.

| Extrinsic (most common) | Intrinsic | |
	Intraluminal (rare)	Intramural (infrequent)
Adhesions	Milk curd obstruction	Neonatal atresia
Hernias	Inspissated meconium	Intussusception
External	Foreign body	Small bowel neoplasms
Internal	Worms (Ascaris lumbricoides)	Primary – lipoma, leiomyoma, carcinoid, lymphoma, adenocarcinoma
Incisional	Bezoar	
Metastatic cancer	Gallstone	
Volvulus	Small bowel tumors	Metastatic – melanoma
Intraabdominal abscess		Hematoma
Intraabdominal hematoma		Trauma
Intraabdominal drain		Anticoagulant overdose
Tight fascial stoma opening		Stricture
		Radiation enteritis
		Crohn's disease
		Tuberculosis
		Complication of surgical anastomosis
		Potassium tablets, NSAIDs

segment becomes compromised, leading to ischemia and bowel necrosis. The small bowel, unlike the large bowel, perforates rarely when obstructed – and most often in cases of radiation enteritis or metastatic neoplasms.

Note: In parts of Europe, the term ileus is applied both to a mechanical obstruction and to atony of the bowel related to abdominal surgery or peritonitis; however, in most English-speaking countries, the term obstruction is reserved for the mechanical blockage arising from a structural abnormality that presents a physical barrier to the progression of gut contents. The term ileus probably should be reserved for the paralytic or functional obstruction.

Pathophysiology

Whatever the site and cause, SBO leads to rapid accumulation of luminal secretions, swallowed air, and gas from bacterial fermentation in the bowel segment proximal to the obstruction which becomes increasingly distended. Bacterial overgrowth, bowel edema, and loss of absorptive function follow, enhancing the third spacing of fluid, electrolytes, and proteins into the intestinal lumen. The overall effect is progressive dehydration, electrolyte imbalance, and systemic toxicity. Copious vomiting exacerbates fluid loss and electrolytic depletion. If the condition is not treated promptly, ischemia and necrosis of the small intestine may occur. Obstructed small bowel, unlike the large one, perforates rarely and this is usually due to compromised intestinal wall in cases of radiation enteritis or metastases.

Clinical Presentation

The most common symptoms of SBO are abdominal pain, vomiting, abdominal distension, and obstipation (Fig. 1.1). Abdominal pain is the leading and most constant symptom. In simple SBO, the accompanying symptoms include peri-umbilical and intermittent pain and cramps, that waxes and wanes over 1 to 3 min intervals. It is believed that progression from a colicky to persistent, steady pain is a sign of impending strangulation. In general, pain increases in severity and depth as obstruction progresses. Distension, nausea, and vomiting usually develop after pain has already been existent for some time. In general, the more proximal the level of obstruction,

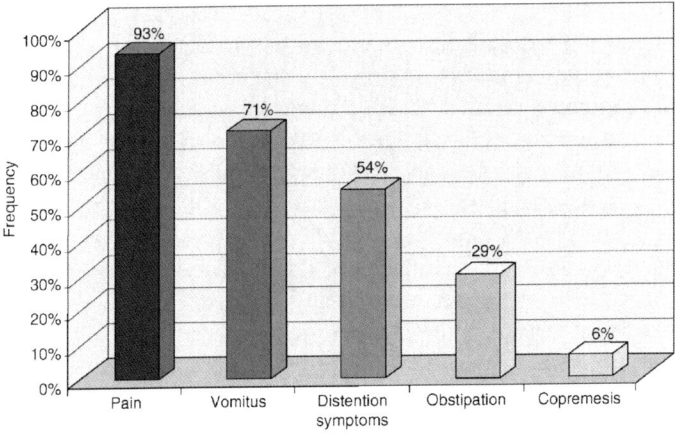

FIGURE 1.1. Frequency of the leading symptoms of small bowel obstruction (Modified from Uhl W et al., 1998. With permission).

the less the distension and the more rapid the onset of nausea and vomiting. Conversely, in patients with distal SBO, central abdominal distention may be marked, but vomiting is usually a late feature. Initially, the vomitus contains gastric juice, which is followed soon by bile, and finally, the vomitus contains feculent small bowel content. Absolute obstipation is a late feature, because the colon requires 12–24 h to empty after the onset of SBO. As a result, flatus and even passage of feces may continue after onset of symptoms. Hypotension, tachycardia, and oliguria correspond to fluid depletion, while tenderness, fever, and leukocytosis suggest strangulation. In the early stages, bowel sounds are usually high-pitched and occur in frequent runs as the bowel contracts to try to overcome the obstruction. A silent tender abdomen suggests perforation or peritonitis and is a late sign.

Diagnosis

A detailed history and a thorough physical examination will provide a correct diagnosis in more than three-quarters of affected patients. The patient should be queried of previous abdominal or pelvic surgery, prior radiation therapy, history of intraabdominal malignancy, inflammation, or trauma, as well as past episodes of bowel obstruction. All medications the patient is taking should be considered as causative, especially anticoagulants. The initial physical examination includes assessment of the patient's vital signs and severity of disease. A nasogastric tube, a urinary catheter, and an intravenous line are placed immediately. The volume and character of gastric aspirate and urine are noted. A full laboratory analysis is routine. The complete blood and chemistry profiles are not helpful in determining the presence or cause of SBO but are useful for the assessment of dehydration and the degree of metabolic derangement. Abdominal examination proceeds from observation to auscultation to palpation and percussion. Abdominal scars, asymmetry, and evidence of peristaltic waves on the abdominal wall should be noted. Auscultation is performed for several minutes – high-pitched bowel tones, tinkles, and rushes are suggestive of an obstruction. Their absence is typical of intestinal paralysis but may also indicate intestinal fatigue and atony from a long-standing obstruction or the development of peritonitis. A meticulous search is made for abdominal wall hernias, especially small inguinal and femoral ones, which are easy to overlook in obese patients. Proper genitourinary and rectal examinations are essential in the search for masses, fecal impaction, mucous, and blood. Patients with an ileostomy should have their stoma examined digitally to make sure there is no obstruction at the level of the fascia. Gentle percussion is performed to search for areas of dullness (suggestive of an underlying mass), tympany (distended bowel loops), and peritoneal irritation. No reliable way exists to differentiate simple from early strangulated obstruction on physical examination, but the more severe clinical course is usually suggestive of strangulation. Serial abdominal examinations are necessary to detect changes early.

An abdominal plain film series is used to confirm the diagnosis of SBO made by history and physical examination. Basic radiologic examination includes an upright chest X-ray to rule out the presence of free subdiaphragmatic air, as well as supine and upright abdominal films. If the patient cannot be placed into an upright position, a left lateral decubitus abdominal film should be obtained. The typical radiologic triad of SBO includes multiple air-fluid levels, small bowel distension, and a paucity of air in the colon and rectal vault (Fig. 1.2). Thickened small bowel loops, mucosal "thumb-printing," pneumatosis intestinals and free peritoneal air are

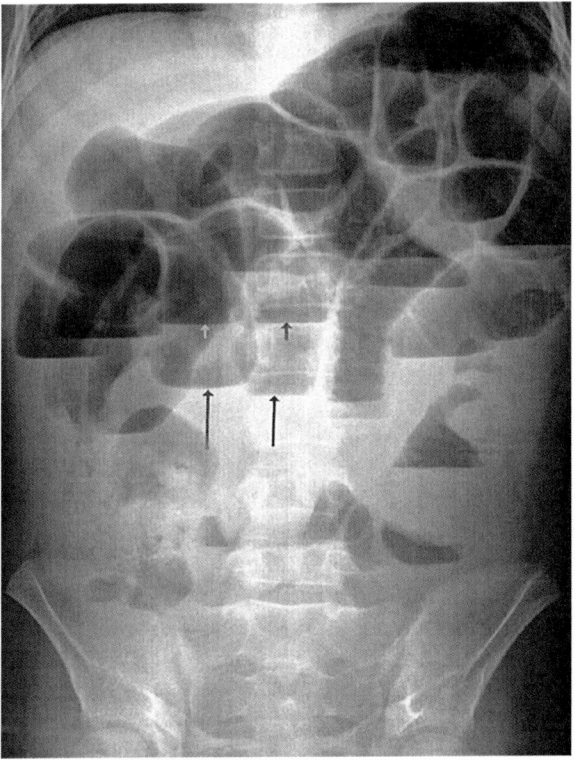

FIGURE 1.2. An upright abdominal x-ray of a patient with distal small bowel obstruction. The arrows indicate well-defined air-fluid levels and distended small bowel loops. Note the characteristic paucity of air in the colon.

considered as evidence of strangulation. It is important to distinguish between small and large bowel gas. Valvulae conniventes are outlined in a distended small bowel and traverse the whole diameter of the bowel lumen. Gas in a distended colon outlines the haustral markings, which cross only part of the bowel lumen and typically interdigitate. Distended small bowel loops usually occupy the central abdomen, whereas distended large bowel loops are seen typically around the periphery. Valvulae conniventes are usually spaced closely and should be within 1–4 mm of each other, but this distance increases with small-bowel distention (the stretch sign). Even when distended, the valvulae conniventes in the jejunum are usually preserved; however, in a distended terminal ileum, they flatten, and the bowel often appears tube-like. Presence of air-fluid differential height in the same small-bowel loop and presence of a mean width greater than 25–30 mm are radiologic signs indicative of a high-grade or complete SBO. When both are absent, a partial SBO is likely or nonexistent. The more distal the obstruction, the more numerous the air-fluid levels. At different heights, the levels reveal a stepladder appearance. An increase in peristaltic activity can give rise to the string-of-beads sign in which the beads represent air trapped within the valvulae conniventes. The coffee-bean sign (a gas-filled loop) may be seen in closed-loop SBO.

A *small bowel follow-through series* and an *enteroclysis* (direct instillation of water-soluble contrast into the small intestine through a tube placed in the duodenum) can reliably and quickly detect SBO and remain the "gold standard" to differentiate partial from complete blockages but are not indicative of the etiology of obstruction. In cases of inconclusive plain films, a contrast-enhanced CT should be the next step in difficult-to-diagnose bowel obstructions. A CT is the study of choice if the patient has fever, tachycardia, localized abdominal pain, and/or leukocytosis. The CT is capable of revealing abscess, inflammatory processes, extraluminal pathology resulting in obstruction, and mesenteric ischemia. It can help to distinguish between ileus and mechanical SBO in postoperative patients and is the preferred method in patients with history of abdominal malignancy. CT rarely, however, shows the source of adhesive obstruction, because it cannot detect adhesions. The diagnosis of obstruction and determining its level is based on the identification of a dilated proximal loop and a collapsed distal loop of small bowel. Bowel wall thickening, portal venous gas, and pneumatosis are CT-signs of early strangulation. Magnetic resonance imaging (MRI) may be used as an alternative to CT in selected patients, e.g., with neoplasms or Crohn's disease; however, this method is complicated, time-consuming, expensive, and not available universally.

Ultrasonography is relatively inexpensive, easy, and quick to perform, but bowel gas and obesity pose problems, and the technique remains operator-dependent. It has no specific role in the diagnosis of an acute SBO but is used widely in the initial investigation of acute abdominal pain. Ultrasonography can often differentiate adynamic ileus of the postoperative state or peritonitis from a mechanical obstruction by depicting peristalsis. This method is preferred in young children, pregnant patients, and as a bedside test for the critically ill. With gallstone ileus, the classic triad of a calcified gallstone in an ectopic position, gas in the biliary tree (pneumobilia), and SBO may be demonstrated. Establishing the diagnosis and cause of SBO should always follow a simple but consistent algorithm in order to avoid mistakes and delay treatment (Fig. 1.3).

Differential Diagnosis

Paralytic ileus, large bowel obstruction, acute pancreatitis, mesenteric infarction, and gastroenteritis should be excluded. Myocardial infarction, intracranial pathology, diabetic ketoacidosis, hyperthyroidism, uremia, and hypokalemia should also be kept in mind. Tricyclic antidepressants and atropine may cause similar symptoms as may peritonitis of any cause. Perhaps the greatest problem arises in the immediate postoperative period after any abdominal

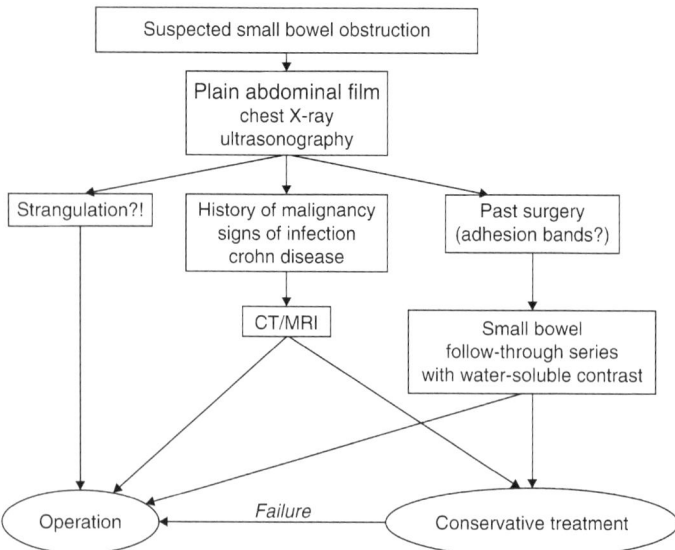

FIGURE 1.3. Diagnostic-treatment algorithm for patients with suspected SBO.

operation, in which it is difficult to determine whether the failure of gastrointestinal function to return to normal is due to a postoperative bowel atony or a mechanical obstruction. In paralytic ileus (a functional disorder seen most commonly after abdominal surgery but also associated with a myriad of acute medical conditions and metabolic derangement), the small bowel is distended throughout its length, and gas is present in the colon on plain films; pain is often not a prominent feature, and auscultation reveals absence of bowel sounds. If there is doubt as to whether a mechanical or functional obstruction exists, a water-soluble contrast study may be helpful. Postoperative ileus usually resolves spontaneously after 4 or 5 days. Intragastric administration of water-soluble contrast may lead to the resolution of this condition in some patients. Figure 1.4 offers a concise algorithm for cases of suspected early postoperative SBO.

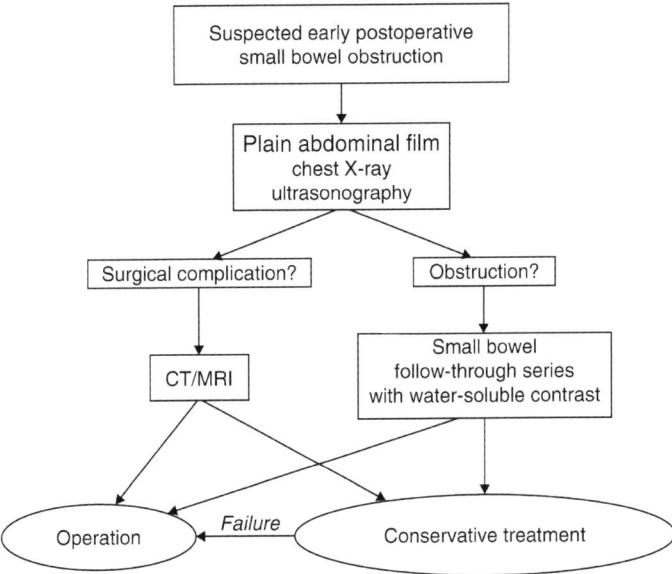

FIGURE 1.4. Diagnostic-treatment algorithm in postoperative patients with suspected SBO.

Treatment

Initial treatment in the emergency department consists of aggressive fluid resuscitation using isotonic saline or lactated Ringer solution, bowel decompression, administration of analgesics, antiemetics, and antibiotic prophylaxis. Fluid resuscitation prior to operation is vital and may require more than 5 l of intravenous crystalloid; a central venous catheter may be preferable. Adequacy of resuscitation is judged by urine output and central venous pressure. Operative exploration in under-resuscitated patients is associated with increased mortality. Oxygen and appropriate monitoring of pulmonary and cardio-circulatory function is necessary. Continued nasogastric suction provides symptomatic relief, prevents aspiration, decreases the need for intraoperative decompression, and benefits all patients. Antibiotics should cover against gram-negative and anaerobic organisms.

A strangulated obstruction is a surgical emergency. A trial of conservatism should be considered carefully in cases of partial obstruction, terminal metastatic intraabdominal malignancy, recurrent adhesive obstruction, and diagnostic doubt about possible ileus in the early postoperative period. Obstructed patients should be observed for no more than 12–24 h and if frequent reassessments show no improvement, the patient should undergo operative exploration. The old rule "never let the sun rise and set on a small bowel obstruction" remains true today.

The nature of SBO determines the type and extent of operative therapy required. While incarcerated inguinal and femoral hernias often allow bowel resection through an inguinal incision, most other cases require exploratory midline laparotomy. A major critical step of the operation is the assessment of viability of the affected bowel segment after relief of the SBO. Any questionably viable bowel should be wrapped in warm, saline-soaked pads and a final assessment made 15–20 min later. Return of normal color, motility, and the presence of mesenteric pulses are signs indicating viability. Alternative but sophisticated and rarely used methods are the intravenous injection of fluorescein with subsequent illumination of the bowel and the standard Doppler ultrasonographic examination or the laser Doppler flowmetry. A resection is the best choice when doubt exists.

Recently, a laparoscopic approach has been used increasingly as a diagnostic and treatment tool for SBO. It is utilized predominantly in cases of adhesive obstruction and requires an experienced team to avoid iatrogenic complications. Experience is essential with laparoscopy, because this technique is not applicable as a standard procedure for SBO unless the surgeon is experienced.

Specific Problems

Intussusception in infants occurs usually in the first year of life and is usually a primary, idiopathic form. The treatment of choice is radiographic reduction with air or barium contrast, with operative treatment reserved for irreducible cases and those complicated with perforation. Adult intussusception is usually secondary and involves a pathologic leading point which is malignant in up to one-half of cases. Thus, most all adults with intussusception require operative exploration.

Patients with SBO secondary to end-stage malignancy present a special therapeutic problem and need highly individual assessment and treatment. When surgery is considered of little therapeutic benefit, continuous nasogastric tube drainage, rehydration, parenteral nutrition, octreotide, antiemetics, opiate analgesics, and comfort measures should be offered.

Early postoperative SBO is defined as that which occurs within 30 days of the initial operation. This condition is difficult to diagnose, because symptoms are often attributed to incisional pain and postoperative ileus. The most common etiology is adhesions; this variant of SBO usually resolves spontaneously within 1–2 weeks as the early formed adhesions undergo a process of spontaneous resolution during this period. This condition is managed safely by nasogastric decompression, and only patients with evidence of strangulation should be operated on expeditiously. Postoperative SBO should be distinguished from postoperative adynamic ileus.

In cases of inflammatory bowel disease, treatment is generally non-operative in combination with high-dose steroids. Parenteral treatment may be considered for prolonged periods of bowel rest. If non-operative treatment fails, resectional surgery of the strictured bowel segment will be necessary.

With radiation enteritis, non-operative treatment accompanied by steroids is usually sufficient in acute postradiation cases. If obstruction is a chronic sequel of radiation therapy, operative intervention is indicated.

Outcome

Complications related to the operative treatment of SBO include anastomotic leakage, sepsis, intraabdominal abscess, postoperative bleeding, wound dehiscence, aspiration, short-bowel syndrome (as a result of multiple resections or massive resection), and death (most often secondary to delayed treatment). Complete obstructions treated successfully non-operatively have a greater incidence of recurrence than those treated surgically.

Mortality and morbidity are dependent on the early recognition and correct diagnosis of obstruction, its etiology, the patient's age and comorbidities at presentation, and on delay in treatment. If untreated, a strangulated SBO causes death in 100% of patients. Thus, early operative intervention is essential. The mortality rate is 25% if the operation is postponed beyond 36 hours. If operation is performed within 36 h, the mortality decreases to 8%. With proper diagnosis and treatment of the obstruction, prognosis is good, and mortality under 3% can be achieved.

Selected Readings

Flasar MH, Goldberg E (2006) Acute abdominal pain. Med Clin N Am 90:481–503

Helton WS (1996) Intestinal obstruction. Chapter 6 in: Wilmore DW, Cheung LY, Harken AH, (eds) et al. SA Surgery CD. Scientific American, New York, pp. 1–22

Khan AN, Howart J (2004) Small-bowel obstruction. http:// www. emedicine.com/radio/topic781.htm

Margenthaler JA, Longo WE, Virgo KS et al. (2006) Risk factors for adverse outcomes following surgery for small bowel obstruction. Ann Surg 243:456–464

Nobie BA, Khalsa SS (2005) Obstruction, small bowel. http://www. emedicine.com/emerg/topic66.htm

Ottinger LW (1995) Small bowel obstruction. In: Morris PJ, Malt RA (eds) Oxford textbook of surgery CD. AND Electronic Publishing B.V/Oxford University Press, Rotterdam/Oxford pp. 961–965

Playforth RH, Holloway JB, Griffen WO (1970) Mechanical small bowel obstruction: a plea for earlier surgical intervention. Ann Surg 171:783–787

Quickel R, Hodin R (2006) Clinical manifestations and diagnosis of small bowel obstruction. Treatment of small bowel obstruction. In: Rose BD (ed) UpToDate 14.1. UpToDate, Watham

Uhl W, Herzog RI, Sadowski C et al. (1998) The surgical treatment of small bowel obstruction. Zentralbl Chir 123:1340–1345

2
Motility Disorders of the Small Bowel

Reginald V.N. Lord and Lelan F. Sillin III

Pearls and Pitfalls

- A mechanical cause of intestinal obstruction should be excluded before the diagnosis of a functional intestinal obstruction is made.
- A thorough history and clinical suspicion are both important in recognizing and diagnosing small intestinal motility disorders.
- Whenever possible, enteral feeding is preferable to parenteral feeding.
- Postoperative ileus is normal, but prolonged ileus is not and needs to be investigated.
- The development of obstipation after apparent resolution of ileus, with passage of flatus or stool, is a sign of mechanical obstruction.
- Patients with intestinal "pseudo-obstruction" can have true, and even complete, non-mechanical bowel obstruction.
- Intestinal pseudo-obstruction may involve either part or all of the gastrointestinal tract.
- If the diagnosis of chronic intestinal pseudo-obstruction is not considered, unnecessary laparotomy is often performed.
- Patients with suspected primary intestinal pseudo-obstruction require very specialized evaluations to diagnose precisely the type of myopathy or neuropathy present.

K.I. Bland et al. (eds.), *Surgery of the Small Bowel*,
DOI: 10.1007/978-1-84996-372-5_2,
© Springer-Verlag London Limited 2011

Introduction

Classification of Small Bowel Motility Disorders

The two types of small bowel motility disorder included here are *paralytic* or *adynamic ileus* and the *chronic small intestinal hypomotility* or *pseudo-obstruction syndromes*. Intestinal pseudo-obstruction syndromes can be either primary or secondary motility disorders, whereas ileus occurs secondary to other pathology. Both pseudo-obstruction and ileus are characterized by abnormally delayed transport of gastrointestinal contents. Postoperative ileus is encountered very frequently by surgeons, unlike the rare chronic intestinal pseudo-obstruction syndromes. Despite promising recent research findings, the difficulty of conducting clinical studies of small intestinal motility means that the complex pathophysiology of both these conditions remains unclear.

Although it may be very difficult to distinguish paralytic ileus or intestinal pseudo-obstruction from mechanical small bowel obstruction due to adhesions, tumor, or other causes, there are important differences in the *typical* features of non-mechanical and mechanical bowel obstructions. These might alert a prudent surgeon and possibly avoid a non-therapeutic celiotomy in patients with pseudo-obstruction.

Paralytic Ileus

Ileus is defined as the temporary loss of gastrointestinal motor function. Ileus thus is an acute, reversible condition that results in a non-mechanical intestinal obstruction. Apart from its almost invariable development after intra-abdominal operations, paralytic ileus can occur after other major operations and after trauma, intra-abdominal or generalized sepsis, myocardial infarction, pneumonia, and electrolyte derangement. A list of causes is shown in Table 2.1. During resolution of ileus, contractile activity usually returns to the small bowel first, followed by the stomach, and only then the large bowel.

TABLE 2.1. Causes of ileus.

Abdominal surgery, especially laparotomy
Major non-abdominal operations
Intra-abdominal infection
Extra-abdominal infection, e.g. systemic sepsis, pneumonia
Peritonitis, e.g. anastomotic leak, bile peritonitis, perforated viscus
Retroperitoneal processes, e.g. pancreatitis, retroperitoneal hemorrhage, ureterolithiasis
Metabolic and electrolyte disturbances, e.g. hypokalemia, hyponatremia, hypomagnesemia, hypophosphatemia
Drugs, e.g. opiates, anticholinergic agents, autonomic blockers, psychotropic agents, general anesthesia
Renal failure
Spinal or orthopedic injury
Diabetic coma
Hypoparathyroidism

The esophagus is not affected. Clinical features of ileus are usually less and may be absent after laparoscopic surgery compared with open abdominal operations.

The pathogenesis of ileus is not well understood. It is not simply a state of hypomotility, as evidenced by the fact that intestinal electrical and mechanical activity usually return rapidly after laparotomy, long before the clinical features of ileus disappear. Loss of both the contractile activity itself and the normal organization of contractile activity are important. Recent studies suggest that important etiologic factors are likely to include recruitment of inflammatory cells to the handled bowel, mast cell degranulation, and activation of inhibitory neural pathways. Also important may be the motilin-related peptide ghrelin, which has been identified as a strong promotility agent in postoperative ileus. Ileal resection and anastomosis results in the early loss, and later partial return, of electrical slow waves and phasic contractions in

muscle near the resection area. This loss of electrical rhyth-
micity is associated with disruption to the network of interstitial cells of Cajal (ICCs), the "pacemaker" cells of the gut.

Clinical Presentation and Diagnosis

The diagnosis of ileus should be considered when signs of
bowel obstruction develop in patients with known causes of
ileus (see Table 2.1).

The clinical features of ileus are abdominal distension,
obstipation, and either vomiting or a large quantity of nasogastric aspirate. Pain is usually absent, but, if present, it is
non-colicky. In the postoperative setting, the pain is usually
no more severe than would be expected with typical postoperative incisional pain and with the associated abdominal
distension. Although the abdomen may be generally tender,
it is usually not localized except at the wound. While the
abdomen is typically silent on auscultation without the groans
and rushes of a mechanical obstruction, tinkles are common,
and a succussion splash may result from the large volume of
fluid contained within the distended stomach or bowel. Plain
erect and supine films of the abdomen show *both* small and
large bowel dilatation with scattered air-fluid levels.

Distinguishing paralytic ileus from mechanical obstruction
in the postoperative period may be difficult but is essential.
Ileus should be managed nonoperatively, whereas mechanical obstruction may require operation, including urgent surgery in some patients. Careful examination and investigation
of patients with continuing signs of obstruction after operation are important in order to detect complications responsible for an ongoing ileus (such as an anastomotic leak) and
to detect mechanical obstruction. Mechanical obstruction in
the early postoperative period may be caused by fibrinous
adhesions or by an internal hernia. Patients with persistent
clinical features of bowel obstruction must be evaluated to
exclude a mechanical obstruction. Passing of flatus or stool,
followed by a return to absolute constipation, may be a sign
that mechanical obstruction has occurred. Similarly, severe

or colicky pain, localized tenderness, radiographic findings of one or more loops of dilated small intestine with a deflated colon, or the absence of gas in the colon is each a sign of mechanical obstruction and not of ileus. Investigation by computed tomography (CT) with luminal contrast or a small bowel follow-through contrast examination may be needed to exclude mechanical obstruction.

Management

The management of ileus in the postoperative period is controversial. The standard treatment has been supportive, with nasogastric decompression, no oral intake, and intravenous fluids until the passage of flatus signifies resolution of ileus. In the absence of strong data showing that nasogastric aspiration reduces the duration of postoperative ileus, there is an increasing trend toward avoidance of nasogastric tubes postoperatively. Similarly, many surgeons now introduce a water or clear liquid diet before the passage of flatus. The management of patients with prolonged postoperative ileus or nonoperative ileus is not controversial. In these patients, the stomach should be decompressed with a nasogastric tube to relieve vomiting and reduce the risk of aspiration. Serum electrolytes should be checked regularly, medications that may induce ileus should be discontinued, and complications such as pneumonia or intra-abdominal sepsis should be excluded and treated aggressively when found. Ileus will resolve spontaneously if the underlying cause(s) is identified and treated successfully. Nutritional support, including TPN, is not usually needed but may be helpful in patients who have both a prolonged ileus and antecedent malnutrition.

There is no convincing evidence that any pharmacologic treatments are beneficial. Attempts to shorten the duration of ileus using prokinetic agents such as acetylcholine, cisapride, motilin, the motilin receptor agonist erythromycin, and other drugs have been disappointing. Cisapride has been reported to be beneficial occasionally, but the use of this drug is associated with a risk of life-threatening cardiac events and is no longer available. Recent studies suggest that effective pharmacologic therapies may be imminent. Promising agents include drugs that block peripheral opioid activity, leukocyte migration, or mast cell degranulation. As well as being a potent gastrokinetic agent, ghrelin also seems to accelerate postoperative small intestinal transit. The identification of the role of an inhibitory neural pathway involving sensory neurons of the lumbar dorsal horn of the spinal cord in the acute phase of postoperative ileus suggests other therapeutic targets. The initial suggestion that chewing gum might be a simple effective treatment for ileus has lost support after a randomized placebo-controlled trial found that chewing gum did not reduce the duration of postoperative ileus.

Intestinal Pseudo-Obstruction

Intestinal pseudo-obstruction is a term applied to a group of rare, incurable conditions that have in common permanent or recurrent hypomotility of either a part or the whole of the gastrointestinal tract. Although in sporadic cases the gut as a whole is abnormal, the most severely affected organ is usually the small intestine. Despite the name "pseudo-obstruction," patients with these conditions after previous abdominal surgery can also have true intestinal obstruction, sometimes requiring total parenteral nutrition (TPN). An increased awareness of these disorders by physicians has resulted in an increase in their recognized prevalence. With the exception of acute colonic pseudo-obstruction (Ogilvie's syndrome), intestinal pseudo-obstruction syndromes are chronic progressive diseases, with subacute and recurrent episodes in most patients that usually progress to chronic, non-resolving pseudo-obstruction.

Physiologically, both the fasted and fed motility patterns are abnormal. Migrating motor complexes (MMCs) are absent or abnormally infrequent during fasting, resulting in stasis, distension, and bacterial overgrowth. Similarly, postprandial motility is either markedly depressed, absent, or poorly coordinated.

The intestinal pseudo-obstruction syndromes are classified as either primary (idiopathic) or as secondary to a known disease. These syndromes are sometimes sub-classified according to whether they have primarily a neuropathic or a myopathic etiology. Familial visceral myopathies and, less frequently, familial neuropathies have both been described, with a clear autosomal inheritance in many myopathic cases. Sporadic idiopathic forms have been termed chronic idiopathic intestinal pseudo-obstruction (CIIP) for the neuropathic patients and nonfamilial hollow visceral myopathy for the myopathic patients. The natural history of CIIP was reported recently in a study of 59 patients followed for a mean 4.6 years. The diagnosis was made a median 8 years after symptom onset and only after most patients had undergone a therapeutic laparotomy for presumed mechanical obstruction. Long-term outcome was poor, and home TPN was needed for almost one third of patients.

A fibrotic myopathy is found in patients in whom the pseudo-obstruction is secondary to connective tissue diseases, with scleroderma being the most common of these disorders. Individuals with myotonic dystrophy, progressive muscular dystrophy, and other muscle diseases have gut involvement but may have few symptoms referable to the alimentary tract. The more common neuropathic causes are diabetes mellitus, hypothyroidism, amyloidosis, and medication use (antidepressants, antipsychotics, anti-Parkinsonian drugs, narcotics, and some antihypertensive and chemotherapeutic agents). Abuse of laxatives, especially those containing anthraquinone, can cause a chronic pseudo-obstruction that effects predominantly the colon. Pseudo-obstruction may also be secondary to a paraneoplastic syndrome.

Clinical Presentation and Diagnosis

Patients with intestinal pseudo-obstruction have a more gradual onset of progressively worsening intestinal obstruction or recurrent symptoms of subacute obstruction. Some patients come to attention only after complete cessation of bowel activity. Common symptoms include abdominal bloating, distension, and discomfort. Patients with colonic involvement may have severe constipation, although diarrhea may also occur as a result of bacterial overgrowth. Involvement of the foregut can cause nausea, vomiting, heartburn, dysphagia, and regurgitation. Children are seen frequently with failure to thrive and weight loss.

Except for those with a known causative disease such as scleroderma, the diagnosis of intestinal pseudo-obstruction is often not suspected or entertained early in its course. As a result, patients with these syndromes undergo exploratory laparotomy frequently to treat a presumed mechanical obstruction, and it is not uncommon for multiple laparotomies to have been performed without the correct diagnosis ever being reached. A careful history, including a detailed family and medication history, should prompt consideration of the diagnosis so that mechanical obstruction can be excluded by radiologic and endoscopic evaluation rather than by operation. The astute clinician may suspect intestinal pseudo-obstruction in the patient without a previous history of abdominal surgery, and thus no adhesions, in whom the clinical presentation is not characteristic of mechanical small bowel obstruction (i.e. slow onset, absence of crampy pain, history of less severe episodes). A slow-growing neoplasm causing a progressive mechanical obstruction may present with similar clinical features and needs to be excluded as does the diagnosis of sprue, which can mimic intestinal obstruction. Radiologic imaging will often show small bowel dilatation, although the diameter can be normal in early or mild cases. Foregut motility studies and gastrointestinal transit studies can be particularly helpful. If a full-thickness biopsy of the small bowel is needed to establish the diagnosis, a laparoscopic approach, in the appropriate setting, is preferred to reduce the risk of subsequent adhesions. The details of the tests used to establish the specific myopathic or neuropathic diagnosis in unclear cases are described in the review by Coulie and Camilleri.

Management

The treatment of known intestinal pseudo-obstruction syndromes is nonoperative. The goals of treatment are to provide nutritional support and improve intestinal motility. Attempts to provide nutritional needs with high calorie, high protein soft or liquid diets are indicated, along with vitamin and mineral supplementation. Antibiotic treatment is used for those with steatorrhea and diarrhea resulting from bacterial overgrowth. Promotility agents, including cisapride (if available), erythromycin, and metoclopramide, may be beneficial in some patients.

In those patients with the most severe myopathic disease and diffuse involvement of the gut, home TPN may be necessary. In patients with less severe disease, enteral feeding may be possible and is almost always preferable to parenteral feeding. Oral feeding can be supplemented or replaced by enteral feeding via a feeding jejunostomy. Surgical resection or bypass is much less effective for these syndromes than it is for isolated colonic hypomotility, but the rare patient with truly localized disease can benefit from resection. Studies of the regeneration of small intestinal motility in an animal model suggest that it may be preferable to construct an end-to-end rather than an end-to-side anastomosis.

Relief of distension and bloating by construction of a venting enterostomy has been reported to reduce the number of hospitalizations, nasogastric intubations, and laparotomies. This operation may even allow some patients to return to enteral feeding. In end-stage disease, small bowel transplantation may be lifesaving.

Selected Readings

Coulie B, Camilleri M (1999) Intestinal pseudo-obstruction. Annu Rev Med 50:37–55

de Jonge WJ, van den Wijngaard RM, The FO et al. (2003) Postoperative ileus is maintained by intestinal immune infiltrates that activate inhibitory neural pathways in mice. Gastroenterology 125:1137–1147

Delaney CP, Weese JL, Hyman NH et al. (2005) Phase III trial of alvi-mopan, a novel, peripherally acting, mu opioid antagonist, for post-operative ileus after major abdominal surgery. Dis Colon Rectum 48:1114–1125

Jones MP, Wessinger S (2006) Small intestinal motility. Curr Opin Gastroenterol 22:111–116

Matros E, Rocha F, Zinner M et al. (2006) Does gum chewing amelio-rate postoperative ileus? Results of a prospective, randomized, placebo-controlled trial. J Am Coll Surg 202:773–778

Murr MM, Sarr MG, Camilleri M (1995) The surgeon's role in the treat-ment of chronic intestinal pseudoobstruction. Am J Gastroenterol 90:2147–2151

Stanghellini V, Cogliandro RF, De Giorgio R et al. (2005) Natural his-tory of chronic idiopathic pseudo-obstruction in adults: a single center study. Clin Gastroenterol Hepatol 3:449–458

Trudel L, Tomasetto C, Rio MC et al. (2002) Ghrelin/ motilin-related peptide is a potent prokinetic to reverse gastric postoperative ileus in the rat. Am J Physiol Gastrointest Liver Physiol 282:G948–G952

3
Appendicitis

Matthew R. Dixon and Michael J. Stamos

Pearls and Pitfalls

- Although symptoms from appendicitis develop most commonly in the right lower quadrant, patients with long appendices or mobile cecums can develop pain throughout the abdomen.
- When treating suspected appendicitis in women, preoperative computed tomography or laparoscopic approach may be of great value given the broader possible differential diagnosis.
- Consider three diagnostic elements separately: history, physical examination, and laboratory/ radiologic investigations. If two of the three support the diagnosis of appendicitis, the patient warrants operative evaluation.
- Computed tomography clearly demonstrating intraluminal contrast filling of the entire appendix excludes the diagnosis of appendicitis.
- Patients with a prolonged history of symptoms or a palpable mass suggestive of contained perforation may be best treated with non-operative management rather than urgent operation.
- The diagnosis of appendicitis can be challenging to establish in pregnant and immunocompromised patients; optimally, operative management should not be delayed in these patient groups.

K.I. Bland et al. (eds.), *Surgery of the Small Bowel*,
DOI: 10.1007/978-1-84996-372-5_3,
© Springer-Verlag London Limited 2011

- Care must be taken to identify with certainty the appendiceal-cecal junction to ensure complete appendectomy. Cecal mobilization may be required.
- Data establishing the role of interval appendectomy following successful nonoperative management of perforated appendicitis is evolving. Interval appendectomy may not be necessary for all patients.

Early Uncomplicated Appendicitis

Presentation

The typical patient with early appendicitis will present with vague periumbilical pain and anorexia during the first 24 h of symptoms. The pathophysiology of appendicitis is due to intraluminal appendiceal obstruction, most commonly from an appendiceal fecolith. Early in the course of the disease, the inflammation is limited to the visceral peritoneum, which does not localize the pain to the source in the right lower quadrant and results, instead, in vague discomfort. Patients may also give a history of nausea or vomiting, but patients with appendicitis usually describe the pain as preceding the nausea and vomiting. When nausea and vomiting occur first, gastroenteritis should be suspected. As the depth of inflammation progresses and begins to involve the parietal peritoneum, patients usually notice that the pain localizes to the right lower quadrant.

Diagnosis

When evaluating patients with appendicitis, it may be useful to consider three elements separately: history, physical examination, and laboratory/radiologic investigations. Many clinicians feel that if a patient has two of the three elements supporting the diagnosis of appendicitis, the patient warrants operative intervention. In addition to the classic history described above, patients with early appendicitis usually have a low-grade fever and mild tachycardia. Abdominal examination will usually demonstrate periumbilical or right lower quadrant tenderness with possible localized peritoneal signs. Pain may be most severe at the McBurney's point, a position two-thirds of the way from the umbilicus to the anterior superior iliac spine. In women, pelvic examination should be performed to exclude pronounced cervical tenderness and to evaluate for possible adnexal pathology.

Patients may have one of the following physical examination findings known to be associated with appendicitis:

- **Rovsing sign** – pain felt in the right lower quadrant on palpation of the left lower quadrant
- **Psoas sign** – pain at the waist with extension of the right hip and leg related to an inflamed pelvic appendix
- **Obturator sign** – pain with flexion and medial rotation of the right leg – related to an inflamed appendix in a pelvic location

Laboratory examination will generally show an increased white cell count with a "left shift". Urinalysis should be performed, although it should be remembered that some red cells in the urine may be found commonly with appendicitis secondary to ureteral inflammation and irritation. Urine B-HCG screen for pregnancy should be performed for all women. The overall differential diagnosis includes urinary tract infection and pyelonephritis, cecal diverticulitis, mesenteric adenitis in children, Crohn's disease involving the distal ileum, and gynecologic causes in women.

Additional work-up and treatment by gender: In several studies, the negative appendectomy rate for presumed appendicitis is substantially lower in men than in women due to the prevalence of gynecologic conditions mimicking appendicitis. Surgeons have accepted historically an overall negative exploration rate of 10% due to diagnostic uncertainty related to appendicitis. With the advent of computed tomography (CT), the ability to establish the diagnosis correctly has improved greatly, and the negative appendectomy rate has been decreased safely. Some authors have suggested that, with appropriate use of CT, the rate may be lowered to less than 2% (Figs. 3.1–3.3). In the past, rectal contrast has been employed to facilitate intraluminal filling of the appendix; however, with the evolution of more sophisticated CT scanners, rectal contrast may not always be necessary.

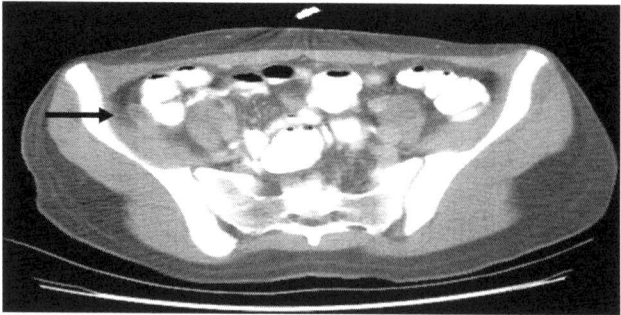

FIGURE 3.1. Retrocecal appendicitis: non contrast-filled thickened appendix (*arrow*) adjacent to iliacus muscle.

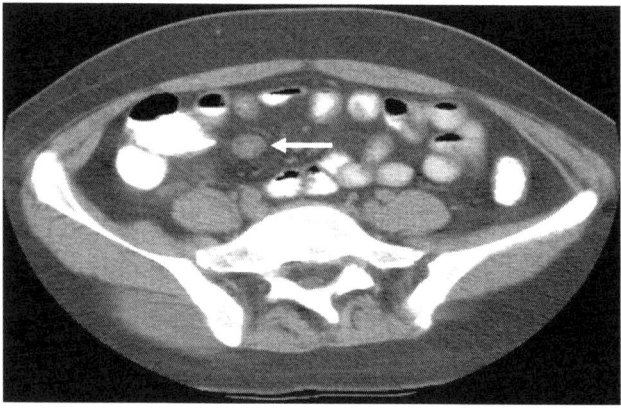

FIGURE 3.2. "Arrowhead sign": note contrast "pointing" to appendiceal orifice, local cecal wall thickening, and thickened appendix medially (*arrow*).

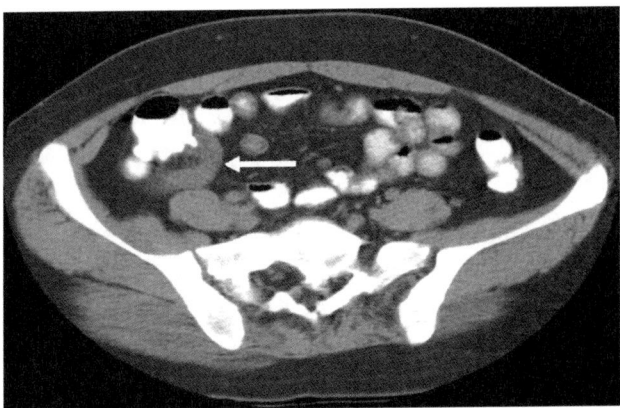

FIGURE 3.3. "Arrowhead sign": note contrast "pointing" to appendiceal orifice with non opacified thickened appendix extending retrocecally (*arrow*).

Moreover, the newest CT scanners may not require any contrast at all. While the authors do not advocate routine CT in all patients, selective liberal use of the CT is appropriate. Additional preoperative work-up suggestions will be discussed separately for men and women.

Male Patients

The differential diagnosis of right lower quadrant pain in otherwise healthy young men is quite limited. As long as the urinalysis does not suggest pyelonephritis, the literature suggests this is one patient group that will not be helped generally by routine CT or other imaging studies when the clinical presentation is consistent with acute appendicitis. These patients may be taken to the operating room without additional work-up. A laparoscopic or open approach may be utilized depending on surgeon preference. For older male patients, for whom the differential diagnosis includes atypical diverticulitis and cancer, CT may be useful in avoiding an unnecessary emergency operation.

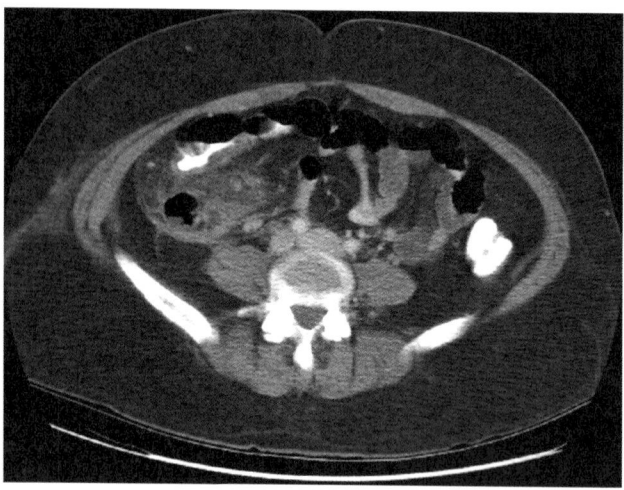

FIGURE 3.4. Advanced perforated appendicitis with extraluminal gas and phlegmon.

Female Patients

Women, particularly those of child-bearing age, presenting with symptoms consistent with appendicitis may actually have symptoms due to a gynecologic etiology such as ovarian torsion, ectopic pregnancy, ruptured luteal corpus cyst, or pelvic inflammatory disease. CT may be useful to confirm the diagnosis of appendicitis prior to operative intervention (Fig. 3.4). Alternatively, a laparoscopic approach may be used, allowing for simultaneous evaluation of the uterus, tubes, and ovaries. In addition to bimanual pelvic examination, pelvic ultrasonography should be considered if the history suggests gynecologic cause, particularly if pelvic inflammatory disease is suspected.

Perforated Appendicitis

Several studies have demonstrated that perforated appendicitis may be suggested by clinical features such as long duration of symptoms (more than 48 h) and higher white cell counts and temperatures.

In the absence of diffuse peritonitis requiring urgent operative management, this patient group may be better investigated with CT to evaluate the degree of perforation and to guide a treatment strategy. CT findings of extraluminal gas, abscess, phlegmon, and wall thickening have been associated with perforation. A rationale underlying the nonoperative management of this group is that patients with long-standing perforation have contained the inflammation and may be treated safely with parenteral antibiotics. Immediate operation for a perforation with significant phlegmon and inflammation may require more extensive resection such as ileocectomy, thereby resulting in higher morbidity. Instead, patients with these findings can be treated with bowel rest, broad-spectrum parenteral antibiotics, and clinical monitoring without immediate operation during the peak of inflammatory response.

When CT demonstrates perforation with abscess, patients may be best treated initially with parenteral antibiotics (Fig. 3.4). It is not necessary to drain all patients who present with an abscess because many periappendiceal abscesses will respond to antibiotic therapy alone, especially those that are multiloculated and/or <5–6 cm in size. Patients failing to improve after 48–72 h may then warrant percutaneous drainage under CT guidance instead of urgent operation.

The advantage gained by nonoperative management for those with the earliest signs of perforation on CT, such as specks of extraluminal gas without evidence of phlegmon, is likely to be more limited and unproven. Patients with an early perforation may be treated by nonoperative management or appendectomy. In contrast, patients with a large phlegmon or palpable mass should be offered conservative treatment initially.

Successful non-operative management of perforated appendicitis is assessed generally by three criteria: improvement in abdominal examination findings, resolution of elevated white cell count as well as body temperature, and ability to tolerate a diet. After successful management of perforated

appendicitis, some authors have advocated interval appendectomy, which may be performed safely using either an open
or laparoscopic approach with minimal morbidity. The data
regarding the benefit obtained from routine interval appendectomy are mixed, because only a minority of patients will
ever experience a recurrence. Some retrospective studies,
including work performed by the authors, have suggested that
recurrent appendicitis develops in a minority of patients and
is likely to be clinically less severe when compared with the
initial presentation. It is important to remember that underlying colonic malignancy is a possible cause of symptoms, and
colonoscopy should be performed in older patients, as well as
those with any clinical features suggestive of malignancy,
including weight loss, change in bowel habits, and anemia.

Appendicitis in the Pregnant Patient

Appendicitis is not an uncommon event during pregnancy
and occurs in approximately 1 in 1,500 pregnancies, making it
the most common surgical condition encountered during
pregnancy. Establishing the diagnosis during pregnancy can
be more difficult and challenging for several reasons. First,
the position of the appendix relative to the abdominal wall
changes as the uterus expands. Therefore, the pain described
during appendicitis in pregnancy assumes a position higher in
the right upper quadrant, which may confuse the diagnosis.
Despite the alleged changes in position, recent studies have
indicated that, in the majority of patients with appendicitis at
any stage of pregnancy, pain occurs within a few centimeters
of McBurney's point. Second, physicians are often less likely
to offer radiologic studies, such as CT, to pregnant patients.
Finally, abdominal discomfort and alterations in appetite may
be a normal feature of late pregnancy, hence, potentially
delaying the diagnosis.

The principle which must be remembered when treating
pregnant patients with possible appendicitis is to avoid perforation, if at all possible. Both maternal and fetal mortality, as

well as the potential for preterm labor, increase substantially with perforated appendicitis.

A collaborative approach with an obstetrician may be useful in decision-making. Graded compression ultrasonography has been considered the first line imaging study. Patients in the second to third trimester may be evaluated safely with CT if the diagnosis is in question after ultrasonographic evaluation. A more difficult situation occurs when patients present in early pregnancy, prior to organogenesis, with possible appendicitis. CT is contraindicated in this group, and operative intervention should be offered liberally. Some have advocated accepting a higher rate of negative appendectomies in pregnant patients given the much higher rate of fetal loss in perforated appendicitis. Magnetic resonance imaging (MRI) has been mentioned in several recent studies as an alternative imaging modality after inconclusive ultrasonography, and may become used more widely for this group in the future when it is readily available.

Several retrospective studies with small numbers of patients have suggested that laparoscopy may be safely performed in pregnancy. In early pregnancy, a laparoscopic approach may be utilized, but this approach may become more difficult in patients late in pregnancy. In the latter, an open approach should be used.

Appendicitis in the Immunocompromised Patient

Diagnosing appendicitis in the immunocompromised patient is much more difficult, because the physical symptoms and clinical signs are usually muted and are more subtle when identified. Immunocompromised patients with right lower quadrant pain also have a much broader differential diagnosis, including viral and fungal colitides, as well as typhlitis in patients receiving chemotherapy. CT may be useful in this patient group to establish a more definitive diagnosis before embarking on an operation. Nonoperative therapy for perforated appendicitis is more dangerous in this population and should probably be reserved for those hemodynamically stable patients with palpable mass.

Operative Approach

Open Versus Laparoscopic Approach

Appendectomy has been performed traditionally with a right lower quadrant, muscle-splitting incision termed the McBurney incision. The muscles are split rather than divided to preserve the integrity of the abdominal wall after closure. A very small incision may be utilized, and the appendix may be found with palpation. On identification, a Babcock clamp is placed on the appendix, taking care to avoid iatrogenic perforation, and the appendix is then delivered through the incision. Cecal mobilization may be required, particularly when the appendix is located in a retrocecal position. Once the appendix is delivered through the incision, the mesoappendix and appendiceal base is divided and ligated between clamps. The appendiceal stump is usually inverted with a purse-string suture at the base. The abdominal wall may be closed in layers with absorbable suture; this closure includes the peritoneum, transversus abdominus, and internal oblique muscles, followed by the external oblique aponeurosis. A midline incision may also be chosen, allowing for extension in cases of widespread inflammation or more extensive surgery.

Laparoscopic approaches have become employed much more commonly. Laparoscopic appendectomy can be performed with three trocar sites after bladder and stomach decompression are achieved with urinary and nasogastric tube placement. One trocar is placed at the umbilicus, a second trocar at the suprapubic position, and a third trocar at the left lower quadrant. One of the trocars should be at least 10–12 mm to accommodate a laparoscopic stapling device (typically placed at the left lower quadrant) and to allow for specimen retrieval. If a 5 mm camera is available, the remaining trocars can be 5 mm. This approach allows the abdominal contents to be evaluated thoroughly before proceeding to appendectomy and provides an outstanding cosmetic result. The patient should be placed in Trendelenberg's position with right-side elevation to optimize appendiceal exposure. Colonic tenia or the distal ileum may be traced distally if the location of the appendix is unclear. Once the appendix is found, it may be grasped and laparoscopic scissors with cautery are then used to allow its full mobilization. Once the cecal-appendiceal junction is found clearly, a window may be created at the base with a laparoscopic dissecting instrument. The window should be large enough to accommodate a laparoscopic stapling device (endoscopic linear cutter). With the appendix retracted anteriorly and superiorly, two consecutive firings of the endoscopic linear cutter – one on the mesoappendix and another at the appendiceal base – complete the operation. A specimen retrieval bag is used to remove the specimen, and the area should be irrigated and checked for hemostasis. The 10–12 mm site can be closed with a laparoscopic fascial closer or closed in the standard fashion; the 5 mm sites require skin closure only.

Perforated Appendicitis

Appendectomy in the setting of perforation may be accomplished by either an open or laparoscopic approach with similar morbidity. Both approaches allow irrigation to be performed successfully and have been associated with similar postoperative complication rates. When operating acutely for perforated appendicitis in the patient with diffuse peritonitis or after failing nonoperative management, extensive inflammation extending to the cecum may be encountered. In these situations, partial or complete ileocectomy may be required. This procedure can be performed expeditiously with a stapling device. The right lower quadrant and pelvis should be irrigated thoroughly. Drains have been used by many surgeons, particularly when an abscess cavity is encountered. The data supporting the use of drains after appendectomy are limited. A recent meta-analysis concluded that drains are indeed harmful and should be omitted. Drain placement should be limited to cases with a large amount of residual inflammatory material after appendectomy and should not be used routinely. Skin incisions associated with conventional laparotomy are usually left open in the setting of perforation, or sutures may be placed to allow delayed primary closure. Skin incisions related to laparoscopic trocar sites may be closed primarily, even in cases of perforated appendicitis.

Selected Readings

Dixon MR, Haukoos JS, Park IU et al. (2003) An assessment of the severity of recurrent appendicitis. Am J Surg 6:718–22

Jones K, Pena AA, Dunn EL et al. (2004) Are negative appendectomies still acceptable? Am J Surg 188:748–754

McGory ML, Zingmond DS, Nanayakkara D et al. (2005) Negative appendectomy rate: influence of CT scans. Am Surg 10:803–808

Oliak D, Sinow R, French S et al. (1999) Computed tomography scanning for the diagnosis of perforated appendicitis. Am Surg 10: 959–964

Oliak D, Yamini D, Udani VM et al. (2000) Can perforated appendicitis be diagnosed preoperatively based on admission factors? J Gastrointest Surg 5:470–474

Pedrosa I, Levine D, Eyvazzadeh AD et al. (2006) MR imaging evaluation of acute appendicitis in pregnancy. Radiology 3:891–899

Petrosky H, Demartines N, Rousson V, Clavien PA (2004) Evidence-based value of prophylactic drainage in gastro-intestinal surgery. Ann Surg 240:1074–1085

4
Short Bowel Syndrome

Jon S. Thompson

Pearls and Pitfalls

- Short bowel syndrome (SBS) occurs after resection of sufficient small bowel to cause nutritional compromise (remnant <120 cm).
- The best treatment is prevention by minimizing the length of resection and preserving all viable small bowel.
- Postoperative management after extensive small bowel resection includes inhibition of hyperacidity, maintenance of fluid and electrolytes, and early enteral nutrition.
- Complication of SBS includes metabolic acidosis, cholelithiasis, nephrolithiasis, bacterial overgrowth, and parenteral nutrition-induced hepatic failure.
- Surgical treatment of SBS may involve restoring continuity and procedures for relieving obstruction or tapering and lengthening the intestine.
- Severe SBS, especially with associated hepatic failure, may best be treated with orthotopic small bowel transplantation.
- Avoid any unnecessary resections; reconstruct rather than resect shortened remnants.
- Avoid hasty decisions to resect reversibly ischemic bowel.
- Minimize extensive resection for inflammatory disease.

K.I. Bland et al. (eds.), *Surgery of the Small Bowel*,
DOI: 10.1007/978-1-84996-372-5_4,
© Springer-Verlag London Limited 2011

- Be certain to document not only the intestine that has been removed, but also the length and site of intestine that remains.
- Anticipating complications is important; consider prophylactic cholecystectomy, avoid blind loops, and prevent irreversible hepatic disease.

Pathophysiology

Short bowel syndrome (SBS) is a clinical condition resulting from extensive intestinal resection and characterized by malabsorption and malnutrition. In adult patients, SBS occurs generally when less than 120 cm of functional intestine remains. Several factors determine the severity and the spectrum of clinical features of the SBS, including the extent and site of the resection, presence of any underlying intestinal disease, the presence or absence of the ileocecal valve, the functional status of the remaining digestive organs, and potential for adaptation of the intestinal remnant. A number of pathophysiologic changes occur in SBS that may cause other specific metabolic problems of importance to the surgeon.

Clinical Presentation

A variety of conditions can lead to SBS. Postoperative complications have emerged as an increasing cause. Mesenteric vascular disease and the treatment of cancer, including radiation therapy, are other intestinal conditions that lead frequently to SBS (Table 4.1). The initial clinical presentation of these patients depends heavily on the underlying diagnosis.

SBS results from a single massive small intestinal resection in approximately three fourths of patients. Patients undergoing massive resection are more likely to be elderly, present emergently, have mesenteric vascular disease, and have a worse nutritional and overall prognosis. One fourth of patients with SBS have multiple, lesser sequential resections. These patients usually have underlying intestinal disease which influences nutritional outcome.

TABLE 4.1. Underlying disease in adult patients with short bowel syndrome

Postoperative resection	52	25%
Cancer/radiation	51	24%
Mesenteric vascular disease	46	22%
Crohn's disease	34	16%
Other benign conditions	27	13%
Total	210	

Preventing the SBS should be the surgeon's first priority. The surgeon should be aware of the need for timely intervention in patients with mesenteric ischemia, early operation for intestinal obstruction to avoid resection, and minimizing resection in patients with underlying chronic, persistent conditions, such as Crohn's disease, that might eventually lead to SBS. Avoiding operation in patients with extensive adhesions or suspected frozen abdomen is also prudent.

Treatment

The appropriate management of patients with SBS, beginning even in the preoperative period, should minimize the predictable complications that might occur and improve prospects for future survival.

Preoperative management: Discussion with the patient and family about the potential consequences of the SBS, including the need for prolonged parenteral nutrition support, should be undertaken before operative decision making whenever possible. There are some patients, e.g., the elderly patient with extensive comorbidity or advanced malignancy, in whom it might be appropriate to consider not resecting diseased bowel that would result in SBS. Obviously, this can be a very difficult decision. For patients who have had previous resections and might predictably require further resection leading to the SBS, there should be greater discussion and consideration of management issues.

The surgeon should try to gain as much information as possible about preexisting anatomy and intestinal disease when considering further operative procedures in patients who have had previous intestinal resection. Contrast-enhanced studies of the intestinal tract are helpful in estimating the residual intestinal length and in assessing the presence of dilation, potential points of obstruction and mucosal disease. Preoperative ultrasonography of the gallbladder should be obtained when appropriate, because patients who have had previous resection are at increased risk for cholelithiasis.

Nutritional status should be assessed so that appropriate nutritional support can be provided during the perioperative period. In patients with acute intestinal conditions likely to require massive resection, management consists of stabilizing the patient hemodynamically and correcting fluid and electrolyte deficits. Preoperative antibiotics should cover colonic bacterial flora. Nasogastric decompression is usually appropriate. If an ostomy is anticipated and time permits, consultation with a stomal therapist and marking the optimal site for the ostomy should be done preoperatively. These stomas often become difficult-to-manage, high-output stomas, and proper construction and positioning are important. Bowel preparation should always be considered when a colon remnant is present, if this is feasible.

Intraoperative management: An important intraoperative strategy is to avoid extensive resection when it is not clearly necessary. Decisions about resection margins and management of intestinal lesions should not be carried out until the entire situation has been assessed fully. It may be appropriate to salvage even a few inches of small intestine in the setting of a severely shortened remnant, despite the potential morbidity of additional anastomoses. Strategies such as stricturoplasty, intestinal tapering, and serosal patching may be helpful in managing specific lesions that would otherwise require resection (Fig. 4.1).

Management of the intestinal disease is an important intraoperative issue. When dealing with intestinal ischemia, any obstruction within or constriction of the mesentery should be relieved, and the bowel should be covered with warm, moist packs and observed for signs of viability. Palpation of pulses and the character of Doppler ultrasonic signals should be used to assess perfusion of the gut wall. Revascularization

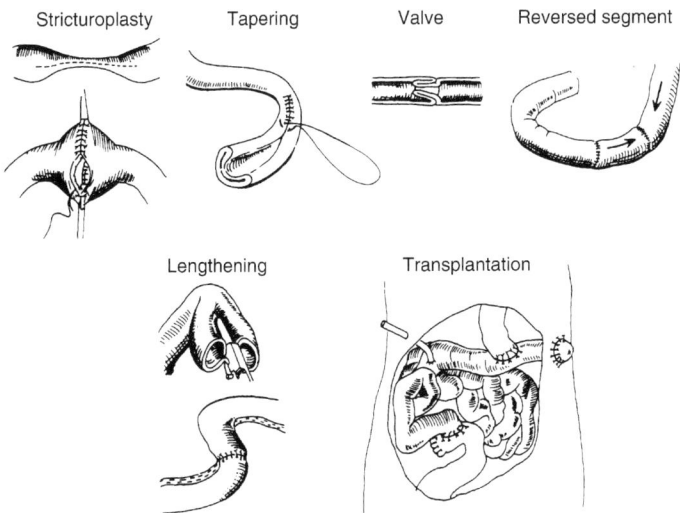

FIGURE 4.1. Operative procedures for improvement of intestinal function in short bowel syndrome (Reprinted from Thompson et al., 1995. With permission).

should be performed if necessary to preserve reversible ischemic bowel. Viability is assessed by improved color, visible mesenteric pulsations, and peristalsis. Intravenous injection of a fluorescent probe with visualization of fluorescent staining and with Wood's lamp to assess diffuse changes and the use of a Doppler ultrasonic flow probe to evaluate blood flow at the margins of the bowel continue to be the most useful modalities. Bowel which is obviously nonviable requires resection; however, when viability is uncertain and recovery of viability is a possibility, a second-look procedure should be considered in retaining questionable bowel.

Intestinal obstruction should be excluded intraoperatively if this possibility has not been adequately assessed preoperatively. This procedure may require passing a balloon-tipped catheter (e.g., Baker's tube or Foley catheter) through the intestinal tract to identify possible stenoses. In patients who already have a short bowel, there may be opportunities to reconstruct the bowel to eliminate blind loops, which can lead to stasis and bacterial overgrowth.

Formation of ostomies may be advisable when the patient is unstable, intestinal viability is questionable, and the patient will be left with a very shortened intestinal remnant, for example less than 90 cm. Duodenal or high jejunal ostomies create difficult management problems. Occasionally, tube decompression is required rather than a stoma. In general, restoring intestinal continuity should be considered strongly whenever distal viable bowel is present.

Because patients with SBS are at increased risk for development of cholelithiasis and acute biliary complications, a prophylactic cholecystectomy should be considered. This decision needs careful evaluation in the patient undergoing a massive resection in an emergent situation. Cholecystectomy would be performed more reasonably in patients who are undergoing elective procedures or who require subsequent reoperation.

Postoperative management: In the early postoperative period, the management of SBS involves primarily the management of the critically ill surgical patient who has undergone an extensive resection. The key issues are control of sepsis, maintenance of fluid and electrolyte balance, and initiation of nutritional support. As the patient recovers, important priorities become maintaining adequate nutritional status, maximizing the absorptive capacity of the remaining intestine, and anticipating and preventing the development of complications related to the SBS and its management.

Total parenteral nutrition (TPN) is usually required for nutritional support during the early postoperative period. Adjustments are necessary for fluid and electrolyte losses, which may be considerable. Most patients require approximately 35 kcal/kg/day and 1–1.5 g protein/kg/day with the appropriate electrolytes, minerals, trace elements, and vitamins. Beginning enteral nutritional support as early as possible once the ileus has resolved is very important, after which the proportion of enteral nutrients should be increased gradually over time. Luminal nutrition maintains intestinal function, maximizes intestinal adaptation, and minimizes complications related to TPN. In general, patients who have more than 180 cm of small intestine remaining will not require TPN or parenteral supplementation for an extensive period. The patients with approximately 90 cm of small intestine, and particularly those who have retained part or all of their colon, especially with an intact ileocecal valve, will require parenteral nutrition for less than 1 year; however, those who have less than 60 cm of small intestine are likely to require permanent TPN.

The transition from parenteral to enteral support requires careful monitoring. The goals are to maintain a stable body weight and prevent large fluctuations in fluid status. Careful monitoring should correct any metabolic abnormalities or nutrient deficiencies. Parenteral nutrition should be decreased gradually as enteral intake increases. A marked increase in gastrointestinal fluid losses in response to enteral feeding usually signifies that increasing the feeding further will not be tolerated. As parenteral requirements diminish, this therapy can be used intermittently until weaning is achieved.

The optimal diet for a patient with the SBS is determined by the length and location of the intestinal remnant, the underlying intestinal disease, and the status of remaining digestive organs. When the remnant is less than 90 cm, a program of more continuous enteral feedings may be necessary to achieve satisfactory nutrient intake. Initially, a high-carbohydrate, high-protein diet is appropriate to maximize absorption. Provision of simple nutrients will keep maldigestion from being a limiting factor during absorption. Fat requires more complex absorptive mechanisms, and stool fat will increase markedly when remnants are less than 60 cm. The initial diet should be hypo-osmolar to minimize gastrointestinal fluid losses, but it may eventually be increased later. Oral rehydration solution will improve absorption in patients with proximal jejunal remnants who are net secretors. If the colon is in continuity, less fat will be tolerated and dietary oxalate will need to be restricted, because the presence of fat malabsorption will lead to an increase in colonic absorption of oxalate with the possibility of renal complications (oxalate stones, oxalate nephropathy). The presence of a stoma may diminish markedly the ability to take in liquids orally due to diarrhea and perianal complications.

Luminal nutrients are important for maximizing the adaptive response of the intestine to resection. The intestinal remnant will increase its surface area and absorptive capacity in the 6–12 months after resection (Fig. 4.2). Provision of fat and

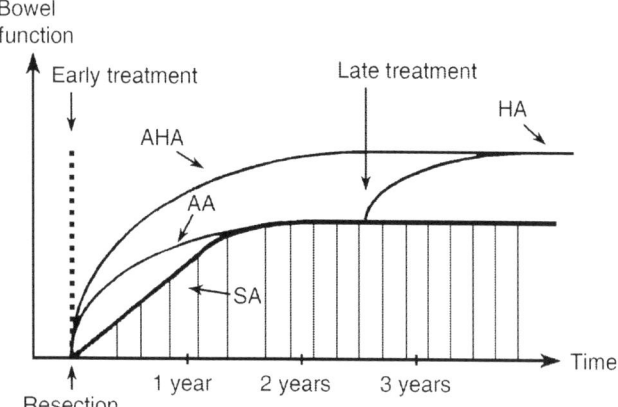

FIGURE 4.2. Schematic presentation of intestinal adaptation. SA: spontaneous adaptation; AA: accelerated adaptation, HA: hyperadaptation; AHA: accelerated hyperadaptation (Reprinted from Jeppesen, 2003. With permission).

dietary fiber may be particularly important in this process. The role of other specific nutrients is currently under investigation. Glutamine is a conditionally essential amino acid that is trophic to the gut. While it is often employed in clinical protocols, its overall importance when given orally still remains unclear.

Growth factors may also stimulate the adaptive response and improve fluid absorption. These agents may accelerate adaptation or produce hyper adaptation (Fig. 4.2). A growth hormone analog has been approved for this purpose. Glucagon-like peptide 2 (GLP-2) is being investigated in clinical trials.

Medical treatment should be directed at minimizing gastrointestinal secretion and controlling diarrhea. Dietary fiber is useful in many patients. Opiates such as codeine, Lomotil (diphenoxylate HCl and atropine sulfate), and loperamide may improve absorption via their antisecretory and antimotility effects. The somatostatin analogue, octreotide, should improve diarrhea, not only by reducing salt and water excretion but also by prolonging small bowel transit time and reducing gastric hypersecretion; however, because of potential side effects and cost, octreotide probably should not be continued indefinitely but rather should be maintained over the time of adaptation (6–12 months). H_2 receptor antagonists and proton pump inhibitors are useful to control the transient gastric hypersecretion and reduce fluid loss, primarily in the first few months after operation. Cholestyramine may be marginally beneficial for binding bile salts and ameliorating the bile salt-induced colonic diarrhea when the colon is in continuity. This approach is most effective when the patient has had an ileal resection of less than 100 cm.

Patients who have had a stoma formed at the time of their resection should be given consideration at a future time for establishing intestinal continuity. There are both advantages and disadvantages to restoring intestinal continuity. By restoring continuity, absorptive capacity may be increased and transit time prolonged. Energy from short-chain fatty acids reaching the colon may increase caloric intake. Having the colon in continuity is equivalent to having another 30 cm of intestine from a functional perspective. There are also psychologic advantages to eliminating the stoma. Furthermore, clinical evidence suggests that infective complications are reduced when the stoma is eliminated. In contrast, however, colonic bile acids may induce diarrhea with associated perianal complications and dietary restrictions. One must weigh the potential of a functional "perianal ileostomy" with intestinal restoration versus a permanent stoma. Patients with colon in continuity are at increased risk for nephrolithiasis. On balance, though, restoration of continuity is generally advisable when more than 90 cm of small intestine is present.

Approximately one half of patients who have SBS will eventually require repeat future intra abdominal operation, most commonly for intestinal complications. In these patients, careful planning should be carried out to avoid further resection. As mentioned previously, utilization of intestinal tapering to improve the function of dilated segments, employing stricturoplasty for strictures, and performing serosal patching for strictures and chronic perforations will help preserve the intestinal remnant. Other intestinal segments that might be recruited into continuity should be identified as well.

Surgical treatment for SBS has several specific goals. One objective is to improve the function of existing intestine by using the strategies mentioned previously. Obstruction should be sought and remedied, ideally by a nonresectional approach. Dilated dysfunctional segments, which may aggravate malabsorption and lead to bacterial overgrowth, should be eliminated (e.g., by tapering enteroplasty). Of note, intestine-lengthening procedures have been utilized in selected patients that permit using dilated segments of bowel to lengthen the intestinal remnant. Both transverse (STEP procedure) and longitudinal (Bianchi procedure) techniques of enteroplasty are often effective and appear to have durable long-term improvement.

Another goal of operative therapy has been to slow intestinal transit and thus improve absorption. This approach has been done with the use of a variety of techniques, including artificial valves and sphincters, reversing intestinal segments, interposing colonic segments in the small intestine, and other innovative approaches. The outcome of these procedures is less predictable, and they should be applied cautiously in carefully selected patients.

The ultimate operative treatment of SBS would be to lengthen the intestinal remnant. With recent improvements in immunosuppression, the outcome of intestinal transplantation is improving. Intestinal transplantation has now become an acceptable clinical approach to this problem in selected patients. Isolated intestinal transplantation is also indicated in patients with loss of vascular access and recurrent sepsis. Combined liver and intestinal transplantation is indicated in patients with irreversible liver failure and SBS.

The appropriate operation for the patient with SBS is determined by several factors, one of the most important of which is the type of nutritional support required. Patients who are able to sustain themselves with enteral nutrition alone should undergo operation only if they demonstrate worsening malabsorption, are at risk for requiring parenteral nutrition, or have overwhelming symptoms related to malabsorption. Patients who require parenteral nutrition but can tolerate a significant amount of enteral feeding may be candidates for operative therapy with the goal being to discontinue

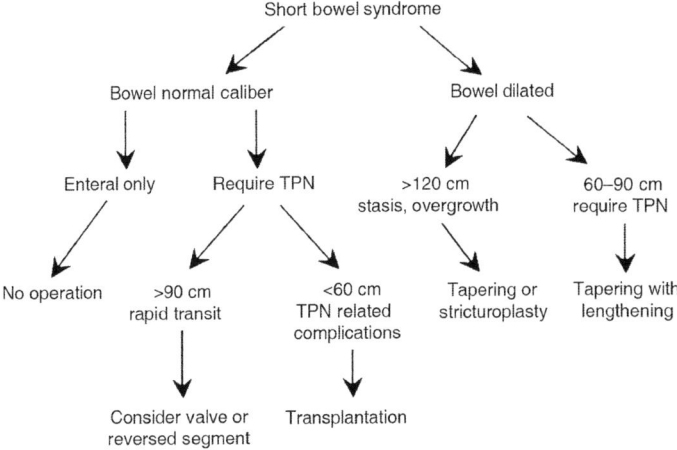

FIGURE 4.3. Operative management of the short bowel syndrome (Reprinted from Thompson et al., 1995. With permission).

parenteral nutrition. Patients who develop significant complications while receiving parenteral nutrition should clearly be considered for operative therapy. Many of these patients, especially when children, will require either combined liver-small bowel transplantation or isolated small bowel transplantation. While liver disease is an obvious indication for transplantation, difficult vascular access and recurrent line sepsis are reasons for considering such therapy. Obviously, other patient-related factors, such as age and underlying disease, will also need to be considered carefully. Thus, the choice of operation for patients can best be tailored in relation to the length of the intestinal remnant, the degree of intestinal function, and the caliber of the intestinal remnant (Fig. 4.3).

Complications

Metabolic complications of metabolic alkalosis and metabolic acidosis (including d-lactic acidosis) are common in patients with SBS related to their tremendous fluid and electrolyte fluxes and the need for specialized nutritional support. Hypocalcemia is commonly related to both impaired absorption and binding by intraluminal fat. Both hyperglycemia and hypoglycemia occur in patients requiring parenteral nutrition. Patients with SBS need to be monitored closely and regularly by a trained nutritionist to detect deficiencies of iron, other minerals, vitamins, and micronutrients.

Symptomatic cholelithiasis occurs in about one third of patients with SBS related to malabsorption of bile acids with the formation lithogenic bile, altered bilirubin metabolism, and biliary stasis. Thus, both pigment and cholesterol stones are found frequently. The natural history of cholelithiasis in this group of patients indicates that they tend to develop more biliary complications and require more complicated operative treatment. Cholelithiasis should always be suspected in patients with abdominal pain and abnormal liver function tests and evaluated with ultrasonography. In patients dependent on parenteral nutrition, intermittent injections of cholecystokinin may prevent stasis and reduce formation of sludge and gallstones. Early enteral nutrition should help reduce the risk of cholelithiasis. The risk of cholelithiasis increases when there is less than 120 cm and small intestine, when parenteral nutrition is required, and when the terminal ileum has been resected. Prophylactic cholecystectomy should be considered in these patients, either at the time of initial resection or at any subsequent laparotomy.

Patients with SBS develop a poorly understood form of gastric hypersecretion in the early postoperative period. This gastric hypersecretion is usually a transient phenomenon and should be treated with medical therapy directed at the increased acid secretion. The need for operative treatment is infrequent, but if required, a procedure such as a highly selective vagotomy may be desirable to avoid gastric resection.

Nephrolithiasis occurs in one third of patient with SBS, related in great part to reduced intraluminal free calcium and the resultant increased absorption of oxalate from the intestine. Because oxalate is absorbed from the colon, this complication occurs primarily in patients with a colon remnant in continuity. Management involves minimizing oxalate in the diet, minimizing intraluminal fat, providing oral calcium supplementation, and maintaining a high urinary volume.

Bacterial overgrowth may be a problem, but it is difficult to diagnose and requires a high degree of suspicion. Bacterial overgrowth decreases the luminal concentration of conjugated bile acids, impairs fat absorption, leads to secretory diarrhea from malabsorbed fatty acids, increases formation of short-chain fatty acids, and results in an increased osmotic load and gas production. It also impairs vitamin B12 absorption. The diarrhea of bacterial overgrowth is primarily a motor abnormality, which can be treated with intermittent antibiotic therapy; however, one should always consider a mechanical cause that may be relieved by operation.

Patient requiring long-term TPN or parenteral supplementation are at risk for catheter-related sepsis and catheter thrombosis, which can limit the clinician's ability to maintain nutritional support in the long term, when available access sites are exhausted. TPN-induced liver disease occurs in approximately 15% of adult patients on chronic TPN. This is a multifactorial problems related to the proportion of enteral calories, overfeeding, and recurrent sepsis. This form of liver disease can be minimized by increasing enteral calories, avoiding overfeeding, using mixed fuels (<30% fat), and eliminating nutrient deficiencies. Administration of ursodeoxycholic acid may also be beneficial. TPN-related liver disease in children with SBS is much more common than in adults and remains poorly understood. Treatment is not very effective and often requires strong consideration of liver-small bowel transplantation.

Outcomes

Permanent intestinal failure is likely in patients with small intestinal remnants less than 90 cm, or less than 30 cm with an intact colon. Permanent intestinal failure should lead to consideration of surgical treatment if severe symptoms or complication occur.

Survival in patients with SBS is approximately 85% at 2 years and 75% at 5 years. An end-jejunostomy, remnant length less than 50 cm, and mesenteric vascular disease have a negative impact on survival. Obviously, survival will also be influenced by patient age, other medical conditions, and underlying malignancy. TPN-induced liver disease has an average survival of only 1 year without transplantation.

Non transplantation procedures for improving intestinal function are successful in approximately 85% of patients. Intestinal lengthening improves intestinal function in 85% of patients early on, but success is less with long term follow up. Success is lowest (50%) in patients who undergo procedures for prolonging intestinal transit time.

One year patient survival after intestinal transplantation is approximately 85%, but decreases to 50% at 5 years. Isolated small intestine, combined liver-small intestine, and multi visceral transplantation (liver, small bowel, pancreas, stomach, colon) all have a role in selected patients. Isolated intestinal transplantation, in general, has a better prognosis than multiple-organ grafts.

Selected Readings

Byrne TA, Willmore DW, Iyer K et al. (2005) Growth hormone, glutamine, and an optimal diet reduces parenteral nutrition in patients with short bowel syndrome. Ann Surg 242:655–661

Chan S, McCowen KC, Bistran BR et al. (1999) Incidence, prognosis, and etiology of end-stage liver disease in patients receiving home total parenteral nutrition. Surgery 126:28

DiBaise JK, Young RJ, Vanderhoot JA et al. (2004) Intestinal rehabilitation and the short bowel syndrome. Parts I and II. Am J Gastro 99:1386–1395, 1823–1832

Grant D, Abu-Elmagd K, Reyes J et al. (2005) 2003 Report of the intestinal transplant registry: a new era has dawned. Ann Surg 241:607–613

Jeppesen PB (2003) Clinical significance of GLP-2 in the short bowel syndrome. J Nutr 133:3721

Messing B, Crenn P, Beau P et al. (1999) Long-term survival and parenteral nutrition dependence in adult patients with the short bowel syndrome. Gastroenterology 117:1043

Thompson JS, Langnas AN, Pinch LW et al. (1995) Surgical approach to the short bowel syndrome. Ann Surg 222:600–607

Thompson JS (2004) Surgical rehabilitations of intestine in short bowel syndrome. Surgery 135:465–470

Thompson JS, DiBaise JK, Iyer KR et al. (2005) Postoperative short bowel syndrome J Am Coll Surg 201:85–89

5
Radiation and Surgery

Mary F. Otterson and Kathleen K. Christians

Pearls and Pitfalls

- Understanding the anatomy of radiation enteropathy is critical in elective cases. Preoperative imaging provides the road map.
- Maximize preoperative nutritional status with enteral (or parenteral) feeding. Micronutrient deficiencies, such as vitamin B 12, may infer the degree of intestinal damage.
- Bowel prep the patient prior to the procedure if possible, because strictures in the small intestine predispose to proximal intestinal bacterial overgrowth.
- Protect normal structures such as the ureter with ureteral stenting.
- Bypass the affected area if safe resection is not possible.
- Consider tissue transfer (plastic surgery) for difficult-to-heal wounds.

Introduction

Whether radiation exposure is therapeutic, accidental, or belligerent, the potentially profound effects produced by radiation alter the outcome of operative interventions. With an understanding of both normal tissue and oncologic radiobiology,

K.I. Bland et al. (eds.), *Surgery of the Small Bowel*,
DOI: 10.1007/978-1-84996-372-5_5,
© Springer-Verlag London Limited 2011

the surgeon is both better able to make informed decisions regarding the patient who has been exposed and to apply the best procedures intraoperatively to avoid complications.

Gastrointestinal Radiobiology

Radiation effects may be divided into prodromal, acute, and late effects of radiation. Prodromal effects occur immediately after radiation exposure and prior to the development of acute histologic changes seen with radiation damage. The well-described effects of acute radiation are attributed to depletion of actively proliferating crypt cells and are associated with profound changes in absorption and secretion. Late effects of radiation are secondary to a combination of ischemic changes and fibrosis.

Within hours of a significant dose of radiation (approximately 400 Centigray [cGy]), prodromal effects of radiation can be detected. These acute symptoms include nausea, vomiting, abdominal cramping, and diarrhea. These effects are due, in part, to the release of serotonin from the enterochromaffin cells of the gut. In animal models (including primates), vomiting is associated with a series of contractions which begin in the mid small bowel and rapidly propel intestinal contents into the stomach immediately prior to emesis. The most striking contraction of this group is the retrograde giant contraction (RGC; Fig. 5.1). The RGC is a powerful contraction that originates in the mid small bowel and rapidly propels intestinal contents proximally into the stomach immediately prior to vomitus expulsion.

Abdominal cramping and diarrhea are associated with the giant migrating contraction (GMC; Fig. 5.2), another type of large amplitude contraction of the small intestine. GMCs are large amplitude contractions that push small intestinal contents into the colon and are associated with abdominal cramping. The GMC may propagate into the colon and, when the contraction reaches the distal colon, is associated with explosive diarrhea. Both Retrograde giant contractions RGCs

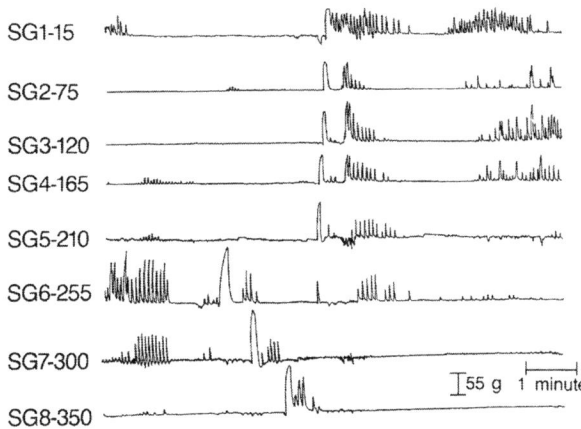

FIGURE 5.1. Both the RGC and GMC originate in the mid small bowel at strain gauge 6. The RGC propagates in a orad direction, propelling intestinal contents rapidly back into the stomach immediately prior to emesis. The numbers listed next to the strain gauge designation refer to the distance from the pylorus in centimeters (Reprinted from Otterson et al., 1988).

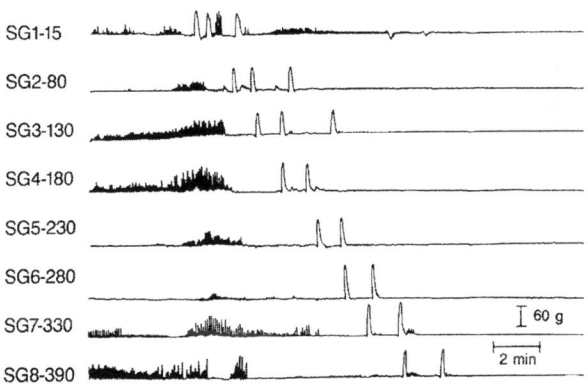

FIGURE 5.2. Three GMCs originate in the duodenum and rapidly propel intestinal contents into the colon. The third GMC does not propagate beyond the mid small bowel at 130 cm distal to the pylorus (Reprinted from Otterson et al., 1988).

and Giant migrating contractions GMCs are associated with radiation therapy but are seldom of concern to the surgeon.

In the case of accidental radiation exposure, the total body dose needed to produce immediate effects of radiation approximates the lethal dose for bone marrow exposure. Thus, in the event of unplanned total body irradiation, vomiting is an indicator that fatal bone marrow suppression may have occurred. Any surgical intervention must proceed with this understanding. Profound bone marrow suppression after surgical intervention for trauma may necessitate exteriorization of intestinal injury as opposed to attempted anastomoses.

The acute effects of radiation are due to the rapid turnover of villous epithelium (5–6 days). Crypt cells are actively dividing cells which, if affected by radiation exposure, do not populate the villi as expected. After fractionated radiotherapy, crypt cell mitoses return to normal within 3 days and villi within 2 weeks of completion of radiotherapy and one can anticipate resolution of symptoms related to mucosal damage soon thereafter. The functional effects of acute phase radiation damage are the diminution of the absorptive capacity of the intestine. Malabsorption of fat, carbohydrates, protein, and bile salts correlate with the morphologic alterations produced by irradiation in small intestinal mucosa. This effect causes a period of reversible nutritional wasting and may produce dehydration. Bile salts are usually efficiently reabsorbed in the distal small intestine. Failure of the small intestinal mucosa results in dumping of primary bile salts into the colon where they are subjected to bacterial degradation. Secondary bile salts thus lead to bile salt-induced diarrhea by acting as cathartics and inhibiting water reabsorption. Expulsion of the watery feces decreases the enterohepatic bile salt pool and causes an increased synthesis of bile salts resulting in choleretic enteropathy. Binding bile salts with cholestyramine or similar agents may alleviate some of the profuse diarrhea that these patients experience. The drug must be within the gastrointestinal tract prior to the first concentrated release of bile.

Lactose intolerance may develop in patients receiving radiotherapy. Mature enterocytes are located at the tips of the villi and provide the enzyme lactase. These cells are missing during radiotherapy and continued ingestion of milk products may exacerbate diarrhea.

Late sequelae of radiation are influenced by the total radiation dose and the volume of bowel irradiated. Symptoms include crampy abdominal pain, bloody diarrhea, tenesmus, and malabsorption of fat and bile salts. Weight loss, obstruction, and occasionally perforation or fistula formation may occur. The area of bowel affected has more to do with bowel exposure than with intrinsic radiosensitivity, i.e., the ileum and rectum are irradiated frequently because they are fixed in position in the pelvis where many disorders treated with radiation therapy occur. The sense of tenesmus may be treated with low doses of tricyclic antidepressants (amitriptyline, 10–25 mg administered at bedtime). Steroid suppositories may also relieve this irritating symptom. Some patients may improve with binding of bile salts using agents such as cholestyramine. Symptomatic relief is key in the management of patients with late sequelae from radiation.

Large vessels exposed to radiation display early vascular spasm which progresses to narrowing, thrombosis, and accelerated atherosclerosis. The microscopic features are obliterative endarteritis, fibrosis, and lymphatic and capillary ectasias. Occasionally, vascular surgical intervention is needed. The advent of minimally invasive stenting techniques may be appropriate, but long term studies in these irradiated patients is not likely to be forthcoming due to their limited numbers.

Patients who have survived cancer, radiation therapy, and chemotherapy often do not approach their next surgical procedure in optimum condition. In elective circumstances, anticipation of intra-operative issues, pre-operative preparation, and fully informed consent are essential. Surgical planning starts with a detailed history and physical examination. During physical assessment, the examiner should look for signs of malnutrition, weight loss, activity tolerance, numbness and tingling of the extremities, or radiation-induced skin changes. The tattoos marking the external focus points for the radiotherapy point to underlying tissue which is likely to be more severely affected. Co-morbid conditions such as diabetes and hypertension suggest accelerated disease processes.

Biochemical and hematologic assessments are helpful. Anemia may reflect subclinical bleeding or persistent bone marrow suppression. With the advent of safe and effective parenteral iron therapy, intravenous iron Dextran, combined with vitamin B12 and erythropoietin, may correct the patient's anemia. Although considered first line for treatment of anemia, oral iron irritates the gastrointestinal tract, and may affect appetite adversely and therefore may not be effective. Many patients find that oral iron therapy worsens their symptoms, resulting in poor compliance.

Along with avoidance of oral iron therapy, elimination of other drugs that produce mucosal damage should be considered. Nonsteroidal anti-inflammatory drugs, aspirin, and bisphosphonates may irritate intestinal mucosa or impede mucosal healing. Alternative therapies or routes of administration should be considered.

Decreased serum albumin is the greatest predictor of morbidity and mortality in the surgical patient. Causes of decreased serum albumin that should be investigated preoperatively include ongoing bleeding, serum loss from the damaged mucosa, malabsorption, and decreased oral intake due to partial small bowel obstruction (SBO). If operation is essential but elective, motivated patients may be able to enhance their nutritional status by sipping supplements to the point of adequate nutritional intake. If adequate nutrition cannot be achieved through oral supplementation, then preoperative total parenteral nutrition (TPN) may be necessary, which allows the patient to receive nourishment at the time of the admission and avoids further nutritional compromise during the postoperative period while awaiting return of bowel function.

Patients with bile salt malabsorption due to chronic radiation changes are at high risk for malabsorption of both fat soluble vitamins and Vitamin B12. Cholestyramine, ½ to 1 scoop first thing in the morning with a possible repeat dose at evening, often decreases the diarrhea experienced by these patients. Either decreased serum vitamin B12 or an increased serum homocysteine level suggests a vitamin B12/folic acid deficiency. Once vitamin B12 deficiency is diagnosed, the patient must understand that therapy will be lifelong. Vitamin B12 deficiency, through increased homocysteine levels, may predispose to premature cardiovascular disease, neuropathy, and gastrointestinal dysfunction.

Patients with sufficient terminal ileal dysfunction to have vitamin B12 deficiency may also have issues with absorption of fat soluble vitamin (vitamins A, D, E, K). Warfarin therapy must be monitored carefully due to its link to vitamin K. Malignancy and radiation damage to venous structures increases rates of deep venous thrombosis (DVT). Routine DVT prophylaxis is therefore recommended perioperatively or for prolonged hospitalization.

Prevention of Radiation Injury

As with many diseases, the best therapy is prevention (Fig. 5.3). Preventing enteric exposure by: (1) performing radiation therapy prior to the operative resection; (2) optimizing positioning the patient during radiation therapy (i.e., prone, with a full bladder to push small intestine out of pelvis); (3) placement of omental flap in the area where radiation will be administered; or (4) placement of Vicryl mesh sling to suspend the intestines from the field of radiotherapy are all worthwhile endeavors.

While described, the placement of tissue expanders is not commonly used to prevent exposure of the normal small and large intestine, probably because subsequent removal usually requires a second operation.

Early Surgery

If operation is planned after radiation, a window of 6–8 weeks post treatment is optimal. This period allows the hyperemic response of radiation to decrease and limits perioperative blood loss. The maximum tumor response to therapy is

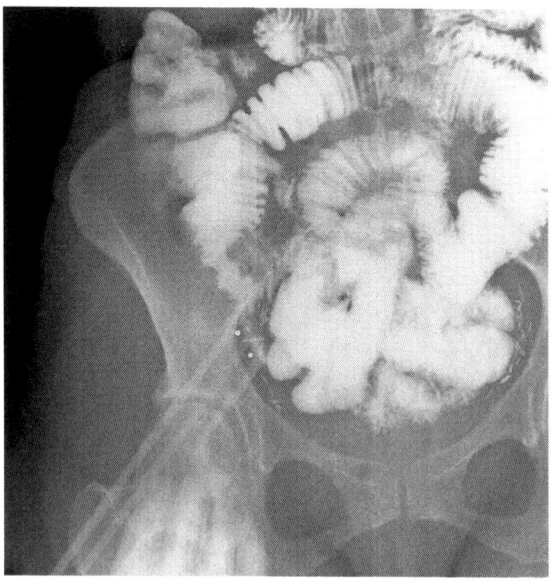

FIGURE 5.3. This x-ray image shows the chronic radiation effects on exposed small bowel adjacent to the area of surgical excision. The patient received both internal and external irradiation for the treatment of uterine cancer.

achieved during this interval. Surrounding tissues, although edematous, have not yet developed the fibrotic scarring and loss of normal tissue planes that characterize the late effects of radiation. Timing is key to optimal surgical results.

Late Surgery

Preoperative planning with the participation of subspecialties (urology, plastic surgery) is essential. Repeat pelvic surgery presents many challenges, especially after prior radiation therapy. Careful review of preoperative imaging to identify affected bowel and adjacent structures that may be displaced or adhesed is very important. Special attention should be given to the ureters which can be obscured by scar tissue.

Preoperative ureteral stents can be a valuable addition for ease in identification during dissection and to both avoid and recognize ureteral injury. While the irradiated ureter may function well without injury, the transected irradiated ureter causes major technical difficulty and results in substantial disability for the patient. Involving the urologist during the planning process may help to avoid this unwanted complication.

Recurrent pelvic cancers in an irradiated field that necessitate operative intervention may leave the patient with a large potential space that will not heal. Preoperative consultation with a plastic surgeon can be useful. Gracilis muscle flaps are frequently used to fill in the space caused by an abdominal perineal resection. Use of a rectus muscle flap must be anticipated, because this flap can be thwarted by poorly positioned ostomies, laparoscopic port sites, or drains that interfere with blood supply of the planned flap. Vacuum-assisted wound closure devices may be employed to limit wound size once vascularized tissue is at the base of the wound. Careful multidisciplinary planning prevents the use of ill-thought-out procedures that would interfere with optimal treatment of these complicated patients.

Of the 5–15% of patients who develop chronic radiation enteropathy after abdominal or pelvic radiation, about one third of these patients require surgical intervention. Because of the high morbidity, operative intervention should be reserved for severe injury. These types of injury indications include high-grade obstruction, perforation, hemorrhage, intra-abdominal abscesses, and fistulas. While the timing and choice of operative techniques remain controversial, the goal of operation is limited resection of the entire diseased segment with primary anastomosis between the healthy bowel segments. Due to the diffuse nature of the intestinal injury and difficulty in distinguishing normal and irradiated intestine, limited resection is often difficult to achieve safely. If hemorrhage is not the indication for operation, the bypass may be performed more safely in such patients.

When undertaking operation for treatment of intestinal radiation damage, good surgical principles should be applied. Skin incisions in the field of prior radiation should be avoided.

Adhesiolysis should also be avoided as it leads to further impairment of an already compromised blood supply and leads to increased risks of perforation and fistula. Whenever possible, anastomoses should be made between segments that are free of disease and with adequate blood supply, even should it require removal of a more generous length of involved bowel. This decision is often the most difficult. Anastomoses involving irradiated segments have leak rates as high as 50%. Distinguishing between normal and diseased segments of intestine is nearly impossible by gross intraoperative inspection, and while incompletely reliable, frozen section analysis of the margins may be helpful. The omentum may be incorporated at the anastomotic site to try to decrease the risk for leak. The surgeon should be prepared to perform an intestinal bypass rather than resection in an unfavorable abdomen.

Disabling symptoms associated with defecation or bleeding should be managed medically prior to any attempt at surgical correction. Formalin application to bleeding sites in chronic radiation proctitis is successful in greater than 80% of patients. A gauze pad soaked with 4% solution is applied to the affected rectum through a proctoscope for 2–3 min until the bleeding ceases. Care is taken to protect normal skin and tissue. Formalin installation (50 ml of Formalin for 30 s, total of 400–500 ml per session) with the placement of a balloon catheter cephalad to the treatment region to protect normal tissue with installation is also successful in 1 in 3 applications. Hyperbaric oxygen has 50–60% success rates in small retrospective studies. The disadvantage of hyperbaric oxygen remains its expense as well as limited access to this therapy.

Endoscopic management using both Nd:YAG laser or argon plasma coagulation for the control of hemorrhage has also been reported. The advantage of argon plasma coagulation is its availability, lesser expense, and limited tissue penetration (2–3 mm). The charred tissue produced by the argon coagulate interrupts current passing through the tissue, while the Nd:YAG laser energy continues to penetrate tissue until it is turned off. Complications of Nd:YAG laser include tenesmus, rectal stenosis, abdominal pain, prostatitis, and fistula formation.

Some patients elect or demand diversion of the fecal stream due to symptoms of severe radiation proctitis to provide some relief, especially if the perianal skin is affected. Endoscopy should be used to differentiate irradiated from normal bowel before the planning of the ostomy site. Use of endoscopic tattooing may help the surgeon locate the segment of colon to be utilized. Depending on distal strictures, a mucous fistula may be needed. If at all possible, a functioning, proximal ostomy should be constructed from normal tissue brought through a non-irradiated location of the abdominal wall. If diversion fails and resection of the rectum becomes necessary, the difficulty of this procedure cannot be over-emphasized. Sparing one rectus muscle (no stomas, no port sites, no drain placement) to fill the void left in the pelvis allows utilization of rectus as a vascularized flap into the pelvis. Consultation with a plastic surgeon, a urologist, and possibly a gynecologist should be considered. This type of surgery is best performed at a tertiary center.

Sometimes general surgeons become involved in procedures for urologic radiation damage, often involving fecal diversion for prostate-to-rectum fistulas and conduits for bladder and ureteral obstruction. Planning for this procedure requires imaging of the ureters, bladder, and colon-nearly simultaneously with three dimensional considerations to achieve optimal results for these unfortunate patients. This planning can be achieved with CT reconstruction or with creative fluoroscopic imaging.

Lymphoma can arise in segments of irradiated bowel. Rapidly increasing serum LDH levels suggest this diagnosis. While chemotherapy may treat this disorder, there is risk of transmural disease, and resection of perforated intestine in the setting of radiation enteropathy may be extremely difficult.

Management of Fistulae

Despite maximum preparation, optimum technique, and good perioperative care, some patients develop enteric fistulas. After recurrent malignancy is eliminated as a cause, control and treatment of the fistula is important. Re-operation, especially in the early postoperative time frame, may not be possible or advisable. Control of the fistula to prevent skin breakdown should be the first priority. Control may be accomplished with an ostomy appliance, wound manager, a catheter and drainage bag, or a vacuum-assisted wound closure device. Increasing the resistance of the fistula by increasing the length of the track to the skin in an enterocutaneous fistula may help. One technique to accomplish this involves re-approximating the skin edges around the fistula tract and controlling the fistula with a catheter. Decreasing the volume of effluent may help the fistula to heal; this can be accomplished by decreasing gastric and enteric secretions using proton pump inhibitors and somatostatin analogues. Keeping the patient NPO and initiating TPN may be necessary. A malnourished patient will not heal a fistula.

When the fistula tract has matured, evaluating the fistula with a fluoroscopic water soluble contrast study or a CT sinogram may identify the source of the fistula and determine whether there is a distal obstruction. If a partial distal obstruction exists in the early postoperative period, delay of any definitive procedure for 8–12 weeks is recommended. If there is no distal obstruction, the chances of healing the fistula are improved; hyperbaric oxygen therapy can be tried. Free flaps or omental flaps to provide a non-irradiated blood supply to the source of the fistula may be helpful. If operative intervention is needed, an ostomy may be necessary. Complex cases should probably be transferred to a tertiary referral center because of all the multidisciplinary services required.

Enterovesical fistulas in the setting of radiation damage are suspicious for recurrent malignancy. While relatively common in the case of inflammatory processes, fistulae from radiation damage take years to develop. Repair depends on the source of the fistula and the non-irradiated surrounding tissue.

Patients with enterovaginal fistulas seek surgical intervention less often than one would imagine. The degree of symptoms experienced by the woman is a function of the size of the fistula opening and the liquid content of the bowel movements. If the stool is liquid, bile salts binders (cholestyramine), the use of fiber, or oral opiates to constipate the patient may limit the symptoms. Surgical intervention for a radiation-induced rectovaginal fistula usually requires a diverting ostomy. Resection and repair in an irradiated field is not likely to be successful, particularly if the connection is between the low rectum and vagina because of the thickness of the tissue and the prior radiation. If the fistula is secondary to a loop of small or large intestine adherent to the vaginal cuff, surgical repair is more likely to be successful, because the offending loop of bowel may be resected.

Summary

No surgeon enjoys the prospect of procedures in the irradiated abdomen. Attention to perioperative preparation, medical optimization, and consideration of non-operative treatments and care for the entire patient is absolutely essential. These patients are generally more ill than other individuals but can be helped in many cases with appropriate surgical intervention.

Acknowledgment

Supported by a cooperative agreement with NIAID, AI067734.

Selected Readings

Cotti G et al. (2003) Conservative therapies for hemorrhagic radiation proctitis: a review. Rev Hosp Clin Fac Med Sao Paulo 58:284–292

Galland RB, Spencer J (1986) Surgical management of radiation enteritis. Surgery 99:133–139

Kinsella TJ, Bloomer WD (1980) Tolerance of the intestine to radiation therapy. Surg Gynecol Obstet 151:273–284

Morgan V et al. (2005) Amitriptyline reduces rectal pain related activation of the anterior cingulate cortex in patients with irritable bowel syndrome. Gut 54:601–607

Otterson MF et al. (1992) Effects of fractionated doses of ionizing radiation on colonic motor activity. Am J Physiol 263:G518–526

Otterson MF, Sarna SK, Moulder JE (1988) Effects of fractionated doses of ionizing radiation on small intestinal motor activity. Gastroenterology 95:1249–1257

Plowman PN, Shand WS, Jackson DB (1984) Use of absorbable mesh to displace bowel and avoid radiation enteropathy, during therapy of pelvic Ewing's sarcoma. Hum Toxicol 3:229–237

Rowe GG (1967) Control of tenesmus and diarrhea by cholestyramine administration. Gastroenterology 53:1006

6
Splanchnic Venous Thrombosis

Götz M. Richter and Jens Werner

Pearls and Pitfalls

- Acute splanchnic or mesenteric venous thrombosis is a rare disease accounting for approximately 10% of all abdominal ischemic events.
- The splanchnic venous system represents all intestinal veins which drain ultimately into the portal circulation.
- In acute and subacute mesenteric occlusion, the presence or absence of clinical or laboratory signs of bowel necrosis mainly reflect the status and severity of the disease. Unfortunately, most of the symptoms are nonspecific and overlap with a variety of other abdominal emergencies.
- In chronic mesenteric occlusion, the extent of portal hypertension and its subsequent complications determine the clinical presentation; this holds true for both cirrhosis-related and non cirrhosis-related causes.
- The preoperative diagnosis of splanchnic thrombosis is made very rarely. Often the diagnosis is an unexpected result of imaging tests (mainly CT) for unclear abdominal pathologies.
- Treatment of acute splanchnic venous thrombosis requires immediate anticoagulation. Regional thrombolysis can be achieved via a catheter placed intraoperatively into the mesenteric vein or via a transjugular-intrahepatic porto-systemic stent (TIPS). In cases of local or diffuse peritonitis, patients need immediate laparotomy and bowel resection for irreversible ischemia.

K.I. Bland et al. (eds.), *Surgery of the Small Bowel*,
DOI: 10.1007/978-1-84996-372-5_6,
© Springer-Verlag London Limited 2011

- Chronic mesenteric venous thrombosis is a result of a hypercoagulable state, including protein C, protein S and antithrombin III deficiencies, and Factor V Leiden. Other conditions predisposing to thrombosis include portal hypertension, cirrhosis, pancreatitis, malignancies, and intra-abdominal infections. The underlying diseases should be identified and treated.
- Currently, portosystemic shunt operations are rarely indicated, because interventional radiologic alternatives exist. This approach is especially pertinent in those patients with good hepatic reserve who do not need liver transplantation in the near future. Alternatively, liver transplantation should be considered in those patients in whom cirrhosis is the underlying disease.

Historical Remarks

Acute splanchnic or mesenteric venous thrombosis is a rare but challenging clinical problem among abdominal emergencies. It was first recognized by Elliot in 1885 as a reason for intestinal gangrenous disease. In 1935, Warren and Eberhard were the first to establish the definite distinction between arterial and venous mesenteric thrombosis as causative factors for bowel gangrene. Grendell and Ockner demonstrated in a systematic analysis that mesenteric venous thrombosis accounts for approximately 10% of all abdominal ischemic events. Imaging techniques started to play an important diagnostic role before sonographic identification of splanchnic vascular pathology by B-mode and Doppler ultrasonography was introduced. As soon as helical computed tomography became available widely, the diagnosis of mesenteric, splenic, and portal venous thrombosis was obtained regularly with contrast-enhanced CT during the venous contrast phase. Ever since, several publications on surgical strategies in occlusive mesenteric disease have stressed the role of imaging in decision making and patient selection to improve therapy and outcome for abdominal emergencies and in elective situations. Furthermore, with the development of MRI and MRA, the visualization of normal and pathologic splanchnic vessels became available even in patients with contraindications against iodinated contrast material. The latest achievements to improve contrast and spatial resolution both in CT and MRI have helped to identify congested intestinal wall segments resulting from the lack of venous drainage, while describing correctly the arterial mesenteric vasculature. Using these imaging techniques, better algorithms for clinical management including the indication for conservative versus operative therapy particularly in patients in whom bowel ischemia is not suspected. Historically, symptomatic patients usually underwent laparotomy for suspected transmural necrosis and bowel perforation. With better imaging methods, these conditions are detected much easier or even ruled out without an operation. Furthermore, recent interventional radiologic advances in catheter technology and local pharmacomechanical thrombolysis have added treatment strategies which deal properly with the causative morphologic and hemodynamic problem by reestablishing free mesenteric venous flow.

Chronic splanchnic thrombosis presents with a distinctly different clinical pattern and is a diagnostic and management challenge as compared to acute or subacute forms. In 1988, Warren summarized for the first time the major differences between chronic, non-cirrhotic portal vein occlusion and cirrhosis-associated portal vein occlusion by characterizing the hemodynamic consequences and therapeutic options. In this clinical context, the complications from portal hypertension, such as esophageal or gastric variceal bleeding, play the predominant role. Hence, therapeutic options focus on endoscopic treatment of varices and surgical shunts. Because TIPS requires an patent portal circulation, it is usually not performed in chronic portomesenteric occlusion. Over the last 20 years, some case reports have emerged describing the use TIPS for treating highly focal portal or mesenteric venous occlusions or high grade stenosis in native or post liver transplantation vasculature.

Anatomic Background

The splanchnic venous system is best characterized as the venous tree of all intestinal veins which drain into the portal circulation. Hence, it shows distinct variations of its anatomic organization as compared to the arterial system. The superior and inferior mesenteric artery are completely independent vessels arising from the aorta at separate levels. The inferior mesenteric vein drains into the splenic vein very close to the confluens of the splenic and superior mesenteric vein. Thereby, both mesenteric veins draining the bowel are dependent on each other. In addition, segments of the ascending and descending large bowel have additional, retroperitoneal draining veins which are tributaries to the inferior vena caval circulation. All pancreatic venous vessels drain directly into the portal vein, and the veins of the pancreatic tail drain into the splenic vein. Similarly, almost all gastric veins are tributaries of the portal vein. The vessels from the lesser curvature drain via the coronary vein into the portal vein. Those of the greater curvature of the stomach reach the portal circulation via gastroepiploic veins which drain into the splenic vein. Typically, the veins of one anatomic bowel segment, e.g. ileal or gastric veins, form large, interconnecting loops in the mesentery ensuring a well-collateralized draining system. Furthermore, at the watershed region between the superior and inferior mesenteric venous drainage at the left colonic flexure, there are also venous collaterals that provide venous drainage between these two major intestinal veins. The symptoms of both, the acute and chronic occlusion of splanchnic veins, are dependent heavily on this anatomic background.

Pathogenesis

Besides its clinical presentation, acute and subacute splanchnic venous thrombosis have distinctly different causative factors compared to chronic occlusion. Various attempts have been made to classify and describe the etiology. Because of their similarities in clinical presentation and causative factors, acute and subacute forms of splanchnic venous thrombosis are discussed together and separated from chronic occlusion in this chapter.

In general, the acute and subacute forms represent the thrombotic venous effect of a procoagulant state. Primary and secondary thrombosis have to be discriminated. Primary thrombosis is generated by primary deficits in blood coagulation and imbalances of blood hemostasis, while secondary thrombosis is caused by local (mechanical) distortion of the venous drainage system regardless of the primary location within the portal tributaries. This classification tries to reflect the corresponding severity of the morphologic extent of venous thrombosis and the clinical symptoms. In spontaneous or primary mesenteric occlusion in young women, oral contraceptives play a major etiologic role and should be considered as a major co-factor for primary thrombosis as is smoking. The acute form of the Budd-Chiari syndrome can be considered in the same pathogenetic context, because it might result from the same coagulation disorders as primary splanchnic venous thrombosis alone. The Budd-Chiari syndrome represents an extremely difficult abdominal emergency associated with very high morbidity. A remarkable overlap between primary and secondary thrombosis might be found in patients who present with splanchnic venous occlusion days or weeks after splenectomy. This situation is particularly true in patients in whom splenectomy was performed for treatment of hemotologic disorders. The local venous trauma might add to the coagulation disorder. In addition, splenectomy alone can trigger delayed (total) mesenterico-portal thrombosis. In Table 6.1, the classification of primary and secondary splanchnic venous thrombosis is outlined in detail.

In chronic venous occlusion, the pathogenesis includes a vast variety of acquired and focal mesenteric venous pathologies. A reasonable classification approach is to discriminate between focal, cirrhosis-associated versus non cirrhosis-associated causative factors. This distinction reflects the different hemodynamic baseline of these two disease groups. In non-cirrhosis associated venous thrombosis, local venous infection (sterile and pyogenic), trauma, and tumor invasion play the predominant role for splanchnic venous obstruction. Liver

TABLE 6.1. Causative factors of splanchnic thrombosis.

Primary thrombosis (inherited or acquired prothrombotic conditions)

Factor V Leiden

Protein C deficiency

Protein S deficiency

Prothrombin gene mutations

Antithrombin III deficiency

Antiphospholipid antibody development

Homocystinemia

Pregnancy

Post-pregnancy

Neuroendocrine neoplasms

Endocrine active neoplasm

Polycythemia vera

Essential thrombocythemia

Paroxysmal nocturnal hemoglobinuria

Secondary thrombosis

Inflammatory

   Diverticulitis

   Crohn's disease

   Ulcerative colitis

   Pancreatitis

   Peritonitis

Postoperative

   Splenectomy

   Visceral resections

   Variceal ligation, embolization

TABLE 6.1. (continued)

Trauma

  Blunt abdominal trauma

  Direct pancreatic trauma

  Direct mesenteric root trauma

  Direct duodenal trauma

parenchyma remains normal in cases with umbilical vein infection and subsequent portal vein thrombosis or in patients with pancreatic cancer and local invasion of the major mesenteric veins. Collaterals can develop gradually and maintain hepatopedal flow. By this phenomenon, multivessel thrombosis is prevented. In contrast, in cirrhosis-associated splanchnic thrombosis, both the causative factor and the hemodynamics are different. Thrombosis occurs secondary to long-lasting reversal of portal flow or on the basis of the development of a hepatocellular carcinoma and subsequent portal invasion.

Classification as acute or chronic splanchnic venous thrombosis might be difficult when previously established obstructive venous pathologies associated with portal or mesenteric venous hypertension promote or predispose to occlusion, or if a hypercoagulable state develops for any reason. Splanchnic venous thrombosis is observed frequently in recurrent chronic pancreatitis. In primary and acute splanchnic venous thrombosis, the origin of occlusion is in large mesenteric veins and tends to spread and propagate to smaller veins. It is of utmost importance to identify the functional status of the collateral pathways to provide a rationale for the clinical management by integrating the knowledge about the individual pathogenesis, the local extent of thrombosis, as well as ischemic or portal hypertensive consequences.

Hemodynamics

The simultaneous thrombotic occlusion of the three major splanchnic veins, the superior mesenteric, the splenic, and the portal vein, represents the most dramatic occlusive event in this vascular territory and is induced most frequently by coagulation deficits. Mortality can be as high as 70% due to intestinal congestive ischemia. Because acute onset of splanchnic venous thrombosis prevents the timely development of venous collaterals to relieve the increased intramural pressure within the bowel wall, hemorrhagic necrosis develops. As soon as the three major draining vessels are affected simultaneously, jejunal and ileal segments have no venous drainage and then depend on the mesenteric outflow via retroperitoneal venous connections of the ascending and descending colon and the periduodenal and pancreatic head collaterals. Therefore, bowel necrosis in splanchnic venous thrombosis most often affects distal jejunal and proximal ileal segments. The time course of the occlusion of the three major vessels determines the severity of the clinical course and its complications.

Splanchnic venous thrombosis associated with a coagulation disorder is often located in the small venous vessels and primarily interferes with the intramural drainage from the bowel. The thrombosis propagates downstream to involve the larger vessels. As long as the thrombosis does not involve all of the three vessels simultaneously, there might be time for collaterals to reach substantial size. In such cases of subacute thrombosis, relief of the venous hypertension via collaterals is just enough to prevent hemorrhagic bowel infarction despite the formation of symptoms from the pain of bowel wall congestion and peritoneal irritation. Therefore, from the hemodynamic point of view, it is justified to discriminate a subacute form from an acute form of splanchnic thrombosis. Hence, splanchnic thrombosis secondary to local venous pathologies tends to have a more benign character. In most circumstances, the underlying disease has already allowed the development of collateral hepatopetal flow when unrelated to liver cirrhosis. This conditions holds true for most of the posttraumatic splanchnic venous pathologies, as well as mesenterico-portal occlusions secondary to pancreatitis or pancreatic cancer. Only the Budd-Chiari syndrome plays a different and much more life-threatening role. As long as the portal vein remains open, blood flow out of the liver might be maintained through hepatofugal flow via the coronary vein as the final outflow conduit. Portal occlusion in Budd-Chiari syndrome might occur when portal flow becomes stagnant as a result of the impaired hepatic vein outflow. Subsequently, when portal occlusion occurs in addition to the Budd-Chiari syndrome, no outflow out of the liver exists, and the liver can infarct within hours.

In chronic splanchnic venous occlusion, the hemodynamics are dominated by the sinusoidal liver pressure and the existence of a substantial portosystemic gradient. In liver cirrhosis, the collateral pathways, e.g. gastric or esophageal variceal systems, are essentially hepatofugal, but they require a patent portal vein as the primary conduit. Whenever a condition occurs which destabilizes this balance between intestinal hepatopetal flow toward the portal vein and hepatofugal flow along the (variceal) venous collaterals, the arterial inflow toward the liver determines its functional reserve.

Clinical Presentation

The etiologic factors causing splanchnic venous thrombosis determine its clinical presentation. In the acute and subacute forms, signs of bowel necrosis are the most important features. Unfortunately, most of the symptoms are nonspecific and overlap with a variety of other abdominal emergency conditions. Clinical signs of arterial and venous mesenteric thrombosis are different. Symptoms associated with arterial mesenteric occlusion are much more distinct and predictive of the underlying disease, while clinical symptoms of venous mesenteric occlusion are often nonspecific and non-diagnostic. If acute abdominal pain, local signs of peritonitis, and laboratory findings suspicious of infection are present, venous mesenteric occlusion should be considered in the differential diagnosis. Nevertheless, these symptoms overlap with other inflammatory diseases, including Crohn's disease, acute appendicitis, and others. In the subacute forms of splanchnic venous thrombosis, the leading clinical symptom is abdominal pain, but, pain is again nonspecific, and laboratory findings are mostly inconclusive as well. Therefore, the primary diagnosis is made very rarely. Often it is an unexpected result of imaging (mainly CT) for unclear abdominal complaints. In the acute form, the pain is colicky and located in the middle of the abdomen, because jejunal and ileal loops are involved most frequently. Fever and rebound tenderness are signs of transmural ischemia related to onset of infarction and subsequent complications. However, when subacute splanchnic venous thrombosis develops, the pain might last for a long time without progression to severe abdominal symptoms. In those cases, patients most often seek care several days after onset of symptoms. They report nausea, vomiting, diarrhea, and hematemesis. The most frequent sign in these patients is occult blood with hematochezia present in up to 20%. Sometimes and particularly in the subacute forms, there is postprandial worsening of the pain. In patients presenting with abdominal cramps and bloody diarrhea, the findings might be mistakenly associated with Crohn's disease. Endoscopy is often negative, and only CT and or MRI establish the diagnosis. In very rare cases, the onset of venous occlusion in small venous vessels does not progress to the major conduits and affects only the draining veins of one or only few loops. This small vessel venous thrombosis is often missed even on contrast-enhanced CT. Only the most recent generation of CT with multirow detector systems (16 detector rows and more) appear to provide enough spatial resolution in combination with contrast resolution to establish the diagnosis under such circumstances.

In chronic mesenteric venous occlusion, the extent of portal hypertension and its subsequent complications determine the clinical presentation. This finding holds true both for cirrhosis-related and non cirrhosis-related causes. Therefore, variceal bleeding, congestive gastritis, and ascites are found in both types of splanchnic venous thrombosis, while decreased liver function remains the hallmark of the cirrhosis-associated thrombotic event. In the latter, the functional reserve of the hepatic arterial system will determine worsening or stabilization of the already impaired liver function. In advanced cirrhosis, portal perfusion is reduced dramatically. Occlusion of the portal vein does not necessarily lead to catastrophic loss of liver function in contrast to the acute form of the Budd-Chiari syndrome.

Clinical Management

Acute mesenteric thrombosis: Treatment of acute splanchnic venous thrombosis requires immediate anticoagulation. In the absence of acute peritonitis and if no signs of bowel necrosis are detectable, long-term anticoagulation is the established treatment (Fig. 6.1). In general, anticoagulation should be continued for the rest of the patient's life. In

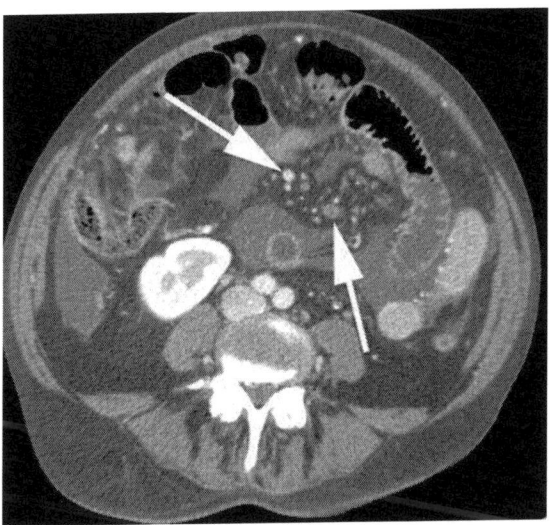

FIGURE 6.1. CT demonstrating a chronic mesenteric vein thrombosis of the jejunum with unaltered flow within the venous branches of the ileum. Conservative treatment with anticoagulation was carried out successfully.

addition, antibiotic treatment as prophylaxis against bacterial translocation should be started as soon as the diagnosis has been confirmed.

Thrombolytic therapy has been advocated either systemically or via an indirect transarterial or direct porto-regional approach. Systemic thrombolysis is associated with the risk of generalized hemorrhagic complications, including intracerebral bleeding and severe intestinal bleeding. Thus, systemic therapy is restricted mainly to heparin treatment. Regional and direct thrombolysis can be achieved via a catheter placed intraoperatively into the mesenteric vein. An adjunctive or alternative technique is direct lysis through a transjugular-intrahepatic porto-systemic stent (TIPS) (Fig. 6.2).

Both techniques allow placement of a catheter in the porto-mesenteric venous system to perform regional thrombolysis with high doses of urokinase or r-TPA and, even more important, over long time periods (up to 20 days). Over the past decade, the interventional catheter placement via TIPS has been often used as the first choice. Operative implantation of the catheter is reserved for those patients in whom the mesenteric veins are thrombosed over a long distance, making it difficult or even impossible to gain safe access transhepatically and for those patients who require immediate operative exploration for bowel infarction. Once an operative approach has been chosen, thrombectomy may be added before the regional thrombolysis via an intravascular catheter. This concept is a therapeutic option as long as the thrombus is not older than 3 days; endothelial cells lining of the mesenteric and portal veins are altered in the region of the thrombus and will be destroyed with subsequent re-thrombosis. Moreover, in most cases, the thrombus will already have extended far into the periphery even in case of timely diagnosis, so that thrombectomy is technically not feasible.

In cases of local or diffuse peritonitis, patients need immediate laparotomy. In those patients, resection of the small bowel and colon which are irreversibly ischemic must be performed with construction of an ileostomy. An anastomosis should be avoided, because progression of the disease cannot

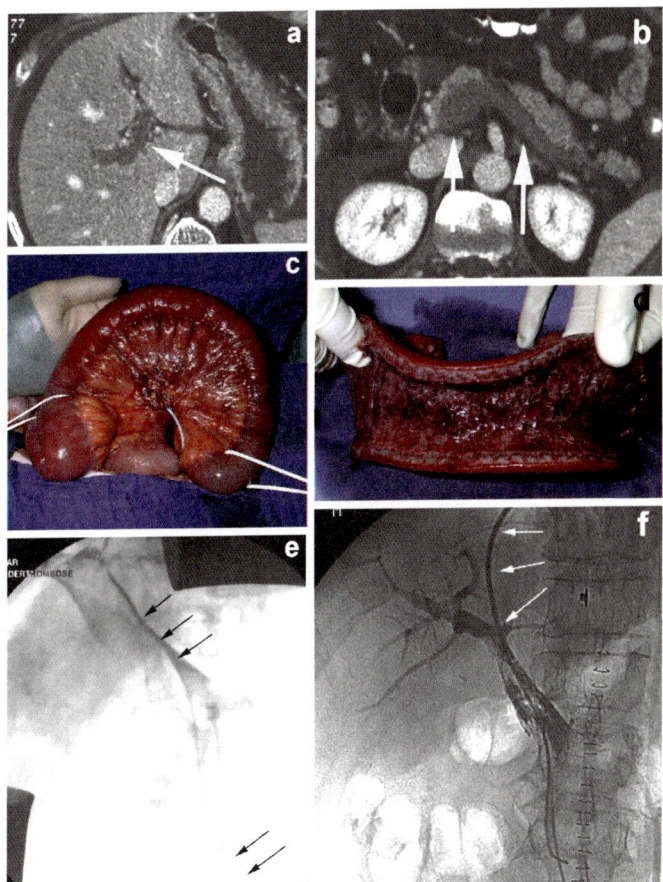

FIGURE 6.2. (**a**) CT showing thrombosis of portal vein without portal vein flow. (**b**) CT demonstrating thrombosis of superior mesenteric vein and splenic vein. (**c**) A catheter was placed into the mesenteric vein for regional thrombolysis. (**d**) The ischemic bowel was resected. (**e**) Mesenteric venography showing the thrombosed superior mesenteric vein and portal vein with the catheter in place. (**f**) TIPS performed for thrombolysis of the portal vein. (**g**) Restored blood flow of the superior mesenteric vein and portal vein after successful thrombolysis. (**h**) Follow-up CT 6 months after thrombolysis demonstrating long-term success of the regional thrombolysis with a patent portal vein.

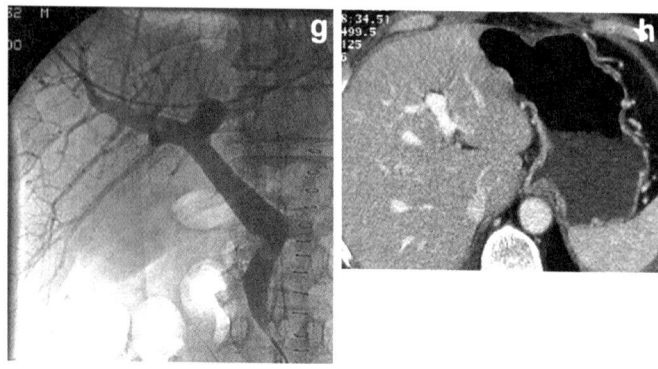

FIGURE 6.2. (continued)

be judged during the first operation but can be observed indirectly by the color of the ileostomy. Additionally, healing of an anastomosis is not guaranteed in ischemic and compromised tissue. If mesenteric venous thrombosis is identified as the underlying cause intraoperatively, a catheter for postoperative local thrombolysis should be inserted into the mesenteric venous system for local thrombolysis. Often, a second look operation is indicated to judge the viability of the remaining gut and by this, the effectiveness of the treatment.

Chronic mesenteric thrombosis: When mesenteric venous thrombosis is identified by imaging techniques, systemic anticoagulation with heparin should be instituted. The patient should undergo evaluation for a hypercoagulable state, including protein C, protein S and antithrombin III deficiencies, and Factor V Leiden. However, other well-known conditions predisposing to thrombosis include portal hypertension, cirrhosis, pancreatitis, malignancies, and intraabdominal infections. The underlying disease should be identified and treated. Emergency laparotomy should only be performed when bowel necrosis or infarction is suspected. In those cases, resection should be performed as described above.

Currently, portosystemic shunt operations are rarely indicated, because interventional radiologic alternatives exist for the treatment of Budd-Chiari syndrome and portal vein thrombosis. This approach is especially true in those patients with Budd-Chiari syndrome with good hepatic reserve who do not need imminent liver transplantation. Alternatively, liver transplantation should be considered in those patients in whom cirrhosis is the underlying disease. The choice between TIPS and a surgical shunt depends on the patient's hepatic reserve and possible timing to transplantation. If transplantation is expected within 1–2 years, TIPS is likely to successfully bridge the patient to liver transplantation without the need for surgical intervention. However, if transplantation is unlikely within 2 years, surgical shunting might be preferred, particularly in younger patients, because TIPS might require more shunt surveillance procedures and subsequent interventions.

Management of **bleeding esophageal varices** has also changed radically over the past decades. Primary treatment is endoscopic variceal sclerotherapy or endoscopic variceal ligation which have low complication rates. Similarly, the minimally invasive nature of TIPS and its successful implementation by interventional radiologists has further reduced the need of surgical shunt operations. TIPS is increasingly used routinely when endoscopic intervention has failed. Liver transplantation is recommended routinely for patients with advanced liver diseases. The time to transplantation is normally bridged with TIPS. Thus, surgical shunts are used more selectively. Surgical shunts are considered in the emergency setting when other modalities, including medical therapy, endoscopic control, or TIPS has failed, in the elective setting as a long-term bridge to liver transplantation, and as a definite treatment approach in patients with noncirrhotic portal hypertension as observed in the Budd-Chiari syndrome. Selective, distal splenorenal shunts are preferred in patients without ascites because of the lower risk of portosystemic encephalopathy. Side-to-side mesenterico or porto-caval shunts have the advantage of relieving ascites by decreasing the intrahepatic sinusoidal pressure and the portal venous pressure gradient.

Selected Readings

Abdu RA, Zakhour BJ, Dallis DJ (1987) Mesenteric venous thrombosis –
    1911 to 1984. Surgery 101:383–388

Bilbao JI, Vivas I, Elduayen B et al. (1999) Limitations of percutaneous
    techniques in the treatment of portal vein thrombosis. Cardiovasc
    Intervent Radiol 22:417–422

Demertzis S, Ringe B, Gulba D et al. (1994) Treatment of portal vein
    thrombosis by thrombectomy and regional thrombolysis. Surgery
    115:389–393

Elliot JW (1895) The operative relief of gangrene of intestine due to
    occlusion of the mesenteric vessels. Ann Surg 21:9–23

Grendell JH, Ockner RK (1982) Mesenteric venous thrombosis.
    Gastroenterology 82:358–372

Kumar S, Sarr MG, Kamath PS (2001) Mesenteric venous thrombosis.
    N Engl J Med 345:1683–1688

Orloff MJ, Orloff MS, Girard B, Orloff SL (2002) Bleeding esophagogas-
    tric varices from extrahepatic portal hypertension: 40 years' experi-
    ence with portal-systemic shunt. J Am Coll Surg 194:717–28;
    discussion 728–730

Slakey DP, Klein AS, Venbrux AC, Cameron JL (2001) Budd-Chiari
    syndrome: current management options. Ann Surg 233:522–527

Warren S, Eberhard TP (1935) Mesenteric venous thrombosis. Surg
    Gynecol Obstet 61:102–121

Warren WD, Henderson JM, Millikan WJ et al. (1988) Management of
    variceal bleeding in patients with noncirrhotic portal vein thrombo-
    sis. Ann Surg 207:623–634

7
Enterocutaneous Fistula

Feza H. Remzi and Victor W. Fazio

Pearls and Pitfalls

- Some 70–90% of enterocutaneous fistulas (ECF) are iatrogenic in origin.
- The management of ECF can be divided into three phases: acute, subacute, and repair with reconstruction.
- The likely presentation and recognition of a postoperative ECF usually occurs 5–10 days after an abdominal operation.
- With early postoperative ECF, fecal diversion with a proximal ileostomy or jejunostomy with or without repair is the procedure of choice, especially with an uncontrolled fistula.
- Note the "window period" before considering any surgical procedure (within 7–12 days from the most recent laparotomy). Within this "window period," severity of adhesions are usually milder, and repeat laparotomy is much easier (unless the first operation involved extensive adhesiolysis, then the window is 1–3 days).
- Initial management of the patient with a new fistula should be directed toward resuscitation and control of ECF drainage by pouching and skin protection; an enterostomal therapy nurse is indispensable.
- Computed tomographic or ultrasound-guided drainage for patients with localized sepsis and PEG tube insertion for small bowel obstruction are important strategies to avoid operation in patients past this window period.

K.I. Bland et al. (eds.), *Surgery of the Small Bowel*,
DOI: 10.1007/978-1-84996-372-5_7,
© Springer-Verlag London Limited 2011

- The subacute phase is the time from the control of sepsis until the time either the ECF heals spontaneously or the decision is made to proceed with repair.
- In the subacute phase, prompt initiation of either parenteral or enteral nutrition therapy is essential.
- Many ECF will close with conservative strategies; if fistula closure has not occurred after 4–6 weeks of nutrition, it is unlikely the fistula will close.
- Definitive repair should be delayed 4–6 months from the date of the initial procedure to allow for softening of adhesions.
- Prior to repair with reconstruction, patients require a complete work-up with nutritional and electrolyte deficiencies corrected, a radiologic road map, and marking by an enterostomal nurse.
- The operation may be a long procedure and may require senior assistance, as well as a multidisciplinary team (urologist, gynecologist, plastic surgeon).
- The goal of the initial phase of the operation is to free all adhesions, drain any remnant abscesses, and relieve any obstructed segment of bowel; leave the ECF management to the last portion of the procedure.
- Resection with anastomosis results in a greater rate of successful ECF closure.
- Consider a temporary high jejunostomy for a period of 3–6 months with parenteral alimentation in patients requiring multiple ECF repairs and residual sepsis.
- The primary aim in closing the abdomen is to provide a biologic cover (skin) over exposed small bowel loops; the expertise of a plastic reconstructive surgeon may be crucial.
- The recovery of these patients is difficult and involves active participation from multidisciplinary teams where the surgeon plays the primary role.
- The surgery of fistula is the surgery for adhesions and understanding the biology of this process – timing is everything.

Enterocutaneous fistula (ECF) involving the small bowel continues to be a challenging problem. Patients are often nutritionally depleted and require meticulous and skilled management to achieve fistula closure. An ECF is defined as an abnormal communication between intestinal lumen and skin. Enterocutaneous fistula may result from one of several conditions. Fully 75–90% of ECF sareiatrogenic in origin (Fig. 7.1) and arise by postoperative leakage from an intestinal anastomosis or from an inadvertent enterotomy during a procedure for inflammatory bowel disease, small bowel obstruction, or operations complicated by severe adhesions or radiation injury requiring extensive adhesiolysis. In contrast, fistulas may be secondary to inflammatory or malignant abnormalities of the bowel wall or from extension from surrounding structures into the bowel wall. The more common intra-abdominal conditions include Crohn's disease, radiation

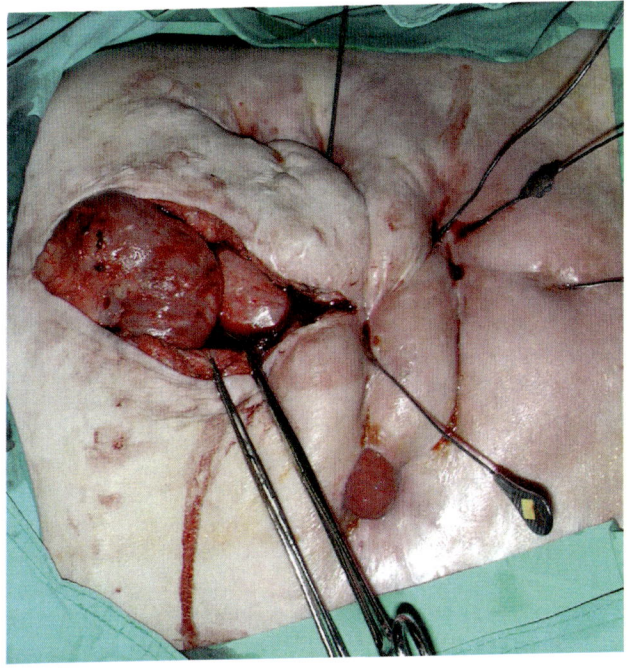

FIGURE 7.1. Complex postoperative enterocutaneous fistula in patient with Crohn's disease.

enteritis, or extension of adjacent disease to normal bowel such as with malignant conditions. When these processes involve the abdominal wall, they can present as a spontaneous enterocutaneous fistula. This chapter focuses primarily on the management of postoperative ECFs; nevertheless, the majority of postoperative and spontaneous fistulas can be managed with the same basic principles of nutritional and surgical treatment despite their differing etiologies.

An ECF is often catastrophic to the health and quality of life of the patient. In the postoperative setting, patients are often septic and malnourished due to surgical stress and ongoing infectious processes. The goals of treatment in the patient with any ECF are closure of the defect and reconstitution of gastrointestinal continuity through an operative or nonoperative approach. Therefore, management of the ECF in the postoperative setting can be divided into three phases; acute, subacute, and repair with reconstruction.

Acute Phase

The presentation and recognition of a postoperative ECF usually occurs 5–10 days after an intraabdominal operation. These patients usually have a prolonged initial recovery with persistent ileus and unknown source of fever; thereafter, the fistula presents with what usually looks like a wound infection, only later noted to be draining enteric content at the time of opening of the wound or after initial wound drainage and packing. With an early postoperative ECF, treatment will depend on the underlying cause, the volume of output (high output generally >500ml vs. low output of <500 ml), time postoperatively, and presumed site of the fistula. Depending on the underlying cause, early reoperation with repair of an anastomotic leak, resection and reanastomosis, or fecal diversion in the form of an ileostomy or jejunostomy may be the procedure of choice. The time interval from the time of initial operation is also critical. It becomes important to note the favorable "window period" before considering any early reoperative procedure. We define this favorable window period as any time within 7–12 days from the most recent laparotomy. Within this favorable window period, the severity of adhesions is usually milder, and a repeat laparotomy with the intent of proximal intestinal diversion and/ or repairing the fistula is justified; caring for a well-matured stoma is much easier than caring for an ECF. This approach will also increase the chance of enteral feeding rather than the need to manage the patient with parenteral nutrition and bowel rest with expectation of spontaneous closure of the ECF. After this window period, we usually defer any attempt of repeat laparotomy provided there is no associated peritonitis or ischemia of the intestine. If re-operation is chosen within or outside this window period, but the surgeon is confronted with a severe obliterative peritonitis precluding a safe adhesiolysis, it would be to the patient's benefit to accept defeat and end any further attempts at adhesiolysis with the intent of coming back at a minimum of 4–6 months later for re-exploration and definitive repair of the ECF, if spontaneous closure fails to occur. Aggressive attempts at complete adhesiolysis in patients with this type of obliterative peritonitis after the index surgery has the risk of further enterotomies, postoperative fistula formation, or worse, an extensive devascularization injury of the small bowel necessitating massive small bowel resection with the possible development of short bowel syndrome. An exception to the 10-day window period involves patients who develop an early ECF after an index operation that involved an extensive adhesiolysis; the favorable time window in these patients may be only 3 days.

The daily volume output of an ECF is also important. The greater the volume, the less chance of closure. An early, postoperative high output fistula suggests a more complete intestinal dehiscence or a distal intestinal obstruction and might precipitate an early re-operation. In contrast, a low output fistula suggests a less complete "diversion" of enteric content and might warrant a conservative, nonoperative approach to management.

Similarly, the presumed site of fistula may also be important. Proximal ECFs are more likely to have high output, less likely to close, will preclude oral feeding, and thus, may warrant a more aggressive operative approach. In contrast, a distal ECF is more likely low output, may allow oral nutrition, and would be more likely to close, depending, of course, on its etiology.

Whether the patient needs a relaparotomy versus a conservative approach, the initial management of the patient with a new ECF should be directed toward a timely and aggressive evaluation and resuscitation. Resuscitation is initiated with crystalloids to restore intravascular volume lost in the fistula drainage. Intravascular deficits may be exacerbated due to sepsis, intestinal obstruction, and edema in the bowel wall. Electrolyte imbalances should be replaced with frequent monitoring of serum electrolytes until stable levels are obtained. These imbalances usually involve potassium, sodium, magnesium, phosphate, calcium, and zinc. In addition to resuscitation, initial management of the ECF should include controlling the fistula drainage by pouching the opening (if possible) and protecting the surrounding skin. Control of the fistula output is often difficult, especially with multiple fistulas or with an open abdomen. An experienced enterostomal nurse therapist is indispensable in the care of the ECF patient during acute and subacute phases of these complex fistula and related wounds. The aim of the wound care is to obtain a pouchable effluent in order to minimize skin excoriation and the frequency of application of the stoma appliance.

Uncontrolled local or generalized sepsis, in association with malnutrition, are crucial determinants of mortality. Percutaneous drainage via computed tomography(CT) or ultrasound guidance is the initial management of choice in patients presenting with an ECF associated with a postoperative intra-abdominal abscess. This drainage may obviate the need for early operative intervention. A definitive procedure can be deferred with the drain left in to control further abscess formation. Aspirated material should be sent for microbiologic culture along with blood, urine, and sputum samples, if appropriate. In most instances, any change in the perioperative course clinically with features of systemic organ dysfunction is due to an undrained septic focus. Thus, prompt investigation an drainage should follow, by bedside ultrasonography or, if the patient is stable enough to be transported, by CT-guided drainage.

In select patients with complex multiple fistulas and an open abdomen who are usually beyond the "window period," pouching of the wound or the fistula alone and control of sepsis may not be possible. Also, re-laparotomy through the initial midline incision with adhesiolysis has the risk of further enterotomy, fistula formation, and devascularization of the small bowel with the possibility of causing a short bowel syndrome. In this group of patients, a left subcostal incision for creation of a high jejunostomy can be life-saving for the control of the chronic recurrent sepsis and may aid in the management of fistula related drainage (Fig. 7.2). We place this diverting stoma as far distally as possible and safe.

Subacute Phase

The subacute phase represents the time period from the control of sepsis until the time when the ECF heals spontaneously or the decision is made to proceed with definitive repair for re-establishment of gastrointestinal continuity. Once sepsis is controlled, initiation of full nutritional support is necessary. The availability of parenteral nutrition has reduced morbidity and mortality by permitting a period of conservative management during which many ECFs can be expected to close spontaneously.

Closure is less likely if the fistula is complicated by inflammatory bowel disease, previous radiation therapy, malignancy, bowel discontinuity with large defects (greater >1 cm2), distal obstruction, short fistula tracts with mucocutaneous continuity, persistent abscess, infection, foreign bodies such as nonabsorbable mesh, or granulomatous diseases/infections.

It is important to calculate accurately the patient's nutritional need to avoid underfeeding or overfeeding. Usually,

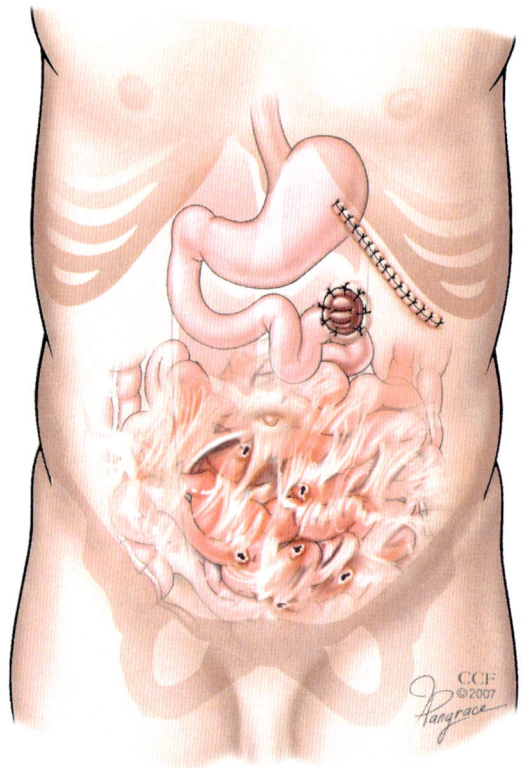

FIGURE 7.2. Creation of diverting high jejunostomy via left subcostal incision in patient with midline hostile abdomen with complex ECF and wound dehiscence.

35–40 kcal/kg/day are required initially in men and 30–35 kcal/kg/day are required in women, but greater caloric requirements may be present if there is ongoing infection, underlying malnutrition, or if the patient has had multisystem trauma. Frequent use of metabolic cart analysis to measure resting energy expenditure can provide a more accurate estimate of caloric needs. The goal of nutritional support in this setting should be achieved with nitrogen equilibrium. The protein requirement of the patient with ECF is at least 1.5 g/kg/day.

In complicated ECFs, consideration should be given to conducting a nitrogen balance study to measure protein needs more accurately.

Regular reassessments of the clinical progress of the patient and laboratory indicators of nutritional status are required to manage the nutritional progress of these patients. Weekly assessment of the transfer in or prealbumin levels is helpful, because these protein concentrations serve as relatively acute phase indicators of the nutritional state of the patient. Parenteral nutrition formulas that will provide a calorie-to-nitrogen ratio of 100:1 to 150:1, while still supplying total caloric and protein needs should be utilized; ideally, 25–40% of total calories can be given as lipids. Fluid requirements for maintenance can be estimated from body surface area and adjusted for existing deficits and ongoing losses from the fistula. Weekly measurements of potassium, magnesium, sodium, and other common electrolytes are useful with supplementation if a deficiency is noted. Ideally, parenteral nutrition should be administered through a single-lumen central catheter.

For patients with a more proximal stoma, fistula output bypasses the majority of the distal small bowel, and this sets the stage for dehydration. The following advice is given to our patients on parenteral nutrition.

- Be aware of added risk factors for dehydration.
- Be aware of symptoms of dehydration – lassitude, fatigue, headache, nausea.
- Maintain intake of adequate oral liquids (if allowed), especially salty soups, electrolyte supplements, etc.
- Avoid high solid fiber/indigestible foods.
- Use liquid loperamide hydrochloride, diphenoxylate hydrochloride with atropine sulfate, liquid codeine, or tincture of opium dosed on a weight basis to thicken enteric output.

The use of somatostatin in the patient with an ECF has received much attention in recent years. Data provide mixed reports as to the overall effectiveness in promoting spontaneous fistula closure. There are data supporting the effectiveness of somatostatin in reducing fistula output, but fistula output does not always correlate with spontaneous closure rates; nevertheless, such decreases in volume and electrolyte losses can make the metabolic and electrolyte changes easier to manage. Therefore, we use somatostatin (100–600 mgm) and its analog octreotide only in patients with high output ECFs in whom the daily fluid requirements and electrolyte imbalance is difficult to regulate.

Early series of managing ECF reported the success of total parenteral nutrition in promoting fistula closure, and thus TPN remains the primary mode of nutritional support in the patient with an ECF to achieve either spontaneous closure or maintain nutritional neutrality until the definitive operative closure. Recent studies, however, have proven that enteral nutrition, when able to be given successfully, has a superior outcome, because it provides the advantages of preserving gastrointestinal mucosa, as well as supporting the immunologic and hormonal functions of the gut and the liver. Enteral feeding also avoids the problem of line sepsis with parenteral feeding. In our experience, we use enteral nutrition whenever possible, especially in patients with low output fistulas(<200 ml/day). For distal ECF, selected "elemental" enteral formulas that deliver pre-digested nutrients (glucose, amino acids, medium chain triglycerides) will minimize fistula output. In contrast, for very proximal ECF, enteral nutrition may be administered distal to the fistula using the residual gut; again, if all the pancreatobiliary secretions are diverted through the fistula, an elemental enteral formula is required unless the fistula output itself is re-administered distally. Although unpleasant and cumbersome, this approach will minimize volume, caloric, electrolyte, and bile salt/cholesterol losses. Nevertheless, while this approach may be the preferred mode of nutritional supplementation in the management of low output fistulas, enteral delivery that is manageable by the patient can be challenging technically, and cumbersome to find and adjust. There is some evidence to support the concept of delivering enteral nutrition at rates unable to supply total caloric needs alone, while still delivering the requisite caloric needs by parenteral nutrition. These lesser rates of enteral calories may maintain gut health and thereby aid recovery.

The fistula wound continues to require special care at this phase, because surgical procedures for permanent closure should not be performed through a septic, indurated, macerated, infected, or denuded abdominal wall. Once again, collaboration by a multidisciplinary approach with enterostomal nursing expertise is important in providing the continual support to these patients, their families, and healthcare workers.

As outlined during the acute and subacute phases of ECF management, strategies for successful resolution of ECF include control of sepsis with imaging-guided drainage and antibiotic therapy, skin protection with stoma care, maintenance of full nutritional supplementation, and fluid and electrolyte balance. In some patients, ECF closure can also be promoted with vacuum-assisted closure systems or fibrin glue, although these techniques have not been evaluated in large series and are not yet approved for this use. While many ECF will close with these conservative strategies, persistent fistulas require definitive surgical intervention. If fistula closure has not occurred after 4–6 weeks of adequate nutritional support and in the absence of sepsis, it is unlikely that fistula will close spontaneously. In most series, 80–90% of the fistulas that eventually close spontaneously will have done so by this time. Therefore, after 6–8 weeks, plans for operative repair should begin.

The timing of repair depends on the clinical situation, presence of multiple adhesions at the time of the original operation, and medical/nutritional state, as described above. This operative repair may involve a major laparotomy and should be delayed to allow resolution of intra-abdominal inflammatory adhesions for patients in the early postoperative phase. The postoperative peritoneal reaction is maximal from the second to tenth postoperative week and maybe exacerbated and complicated by peritonitis or local reaction to the fistula formation. Retrospective studies have shown that mortality is doubled in patients who require re-operation during this subacute time frame of 2–10 weeks postoperatively. In many patients with a complicated ECF, it may be beneficial to delay operative repair of the ECF up to 6 months from the date of the initial procedure. This delay allows for adequate healing of any intraabdominal sepsis and for softening of adhesions, and a much easier operation which will result in a better outcome. An even longer delay may be prudent in patients with a long complicated postoperative course, intraperitoneal sepsis, and malnutrition. Clinical judgement is very important in such a setting.

During this subacute phase until the definitive repair is undertaken, the external drainage of a fistula can become demoralizing and humiliating for the patient. A multidisciplinary approach under the leadership of a surgeon with a trained, enterostomal therapy nurse, parenteral nutrition team, physical and occupational therapist, social worker, and even psychiatrist, are invaluable. Continued reassurance, availability, and affability from the physician will help in this situation. If necessary, psychotropic medications or treatment by psychiatric consulting services are beneficial.

Repair and Reconstructive Phase

Surgery for the definitive repair involves a major laparotomy. The patients and their family should be prepared emotionally and mentally for a prolonged recovery with the potential of recurrence and complications. Therefore, it is imperative that operations to correct an ECF be performed under optimal conditions. Optimal nutritional status and absence of associated sepsis are important parameters that must be obtained prior to definitive operative repair.

Avoiding the Unexpected

Patients need to have complete evaluation with deficiencies corrected whenever possible. The properly prepared patient should have adequate transferrin, prealbumin, hemoglobin, and coagulation levels prior to operation. Diabetes should be controlled, and the patient should not be anemic. Blood should be available, because the majority of these patients have had prior transfusions, and it may be difficult to get proper cross-matched blood at the time of operation if it is needed. Parenteral nutrition should be continued until the date of operation; if a patient is on additional enteral nutrition, this should be stopped 48–72 h beforehand to decrease contamination or associated bowel distention that may complicate the laparotomy.

It is imperative to evaluate these patients fully and be prepared for unexpected findings at the time of definitive operative repair. It is our practice to study every orifice prior to operative repair; trying to dissect out all of the bowel may not be necessary. These tests usually include fistulograms, gastrograffin enemas, small bowel series, and stoma injection. It is imperative to rule out any distal obstruction or associated inflammatory bowel disease or other pathology such as radiation enteritis, malignancy, or granulomatous disease prior to operation. The use of CT is less helpful in delineating site or mucosal details in the evaluation of the fistula patient without sepsis at this stage of the management; in contrast, CT can be valuable in the search for abdominal abscess or associated pathology in the fistula patient prior to definitive surgery. These radiologic studies provide a road map to identify the anatomy and planes and may be crucial to avoid surprises in the operating room. Preoperative marking by an experienced enterostomal nurse is also prudent, even in patients in whom definitive repair is planned. On rare occasions, the repair may be tenuous, and a controlled, well-located proximal loop enterostomy may aid healing of the primary repair and allow an easier, early restoration of full intestinal continuity without the need for a full laparotomy. This loop enterostomy can be taken down by a more localized perisomal approach.

The Operative Repair

The operation may very well be a long procedure. Therefore, the first rule for the surgeon is not to overbook for that day.

It would be important to schedule these complicated cases as the first case and not to schedule any other difficult case for that day. The surgical team should be prepared to obtain assistance from other disciplines such as gynecology, urology, plastics, and any other pertinent reconstructive teams. We usually position the patient in the Lloyd Davis stirrups with arms by the side and shoulder pads for extreme Trendelenburg position, especially for complex cases that involve the deep pelvis. We use ureteric stents liberally to avoid any unrecognized injury and to minimize the time required to identify the ureters during the operation. The availability of lighted retractors is also important. Access to the perineum is often necessary.

Technique of Adhesiolysis and Strategy of Relaparotomy, Repair, and Reconstruction

We begin the operation by entering the abdomen through the easiest place, usually the most cranial part of the abdomen from an area of new or prior midline incision. To accomplish this, we are not hesitant to make a big incision above the umbilicus up to the xyphoid level; the midline incision preserves as much of the abdominal wall as possible for any future stoma, and optimizes exposure and visibility. The goal of the initial phase of the operation is to free all adhesions, drain any remnant abscesses, and relieve all obstructed segments of bowel. Ideally, the entire of length of the small bowel from the ligament of Treitz to the cecum is freed of adhesions. The ECF are left in place until the bowel around them is freed. Our practice is to deliver the matted loops outside the abdomen, decompress the bowel, especially for interloop dissection, and use saline injection with hydro-and extrafascial dissection to avoid an inadvertent injury to the bowel. For hydro-dissection, we use sterile normal saline and a #21 gauge long needle with a 10 ml syringe. The application of saline into the matted loops of small bowel or between the fascia creates a safer plane for sharp dissection and avoids inadvertent enterotomy. Sharp dissection from known to unknown, leaving the most difficult section until last is our usual strategy. Immediate closure of all inadvertent enterotomies and repair of serosal tears will minimize the chance of missing or forgetting to repair these injuries after a long procedure, and avoids further leak with fistula formation in the postoperative period. Successful operation requires the resection of the ECF and associated diseased bowel, usually with a primary, handsewn anastomosis with absorbable sutures. The anastomosis should be distant from the site of any fistula or abscess cavity. In a recent study from our institution, resection with anastomosis resulted in a greater rate of successful ECF closure compared with fistula oversewing or wedge resection. In our past experience, a fistula was oversewn or wedge-resected when it was not thought possible to perform resection due to an inability to adequately mobilize the bowel itself; with this approach, the recurrence rate was unacceptable. If this is the case, or in patients with complex, multiple fistula sites, when the repair is close to any residual sepsis, or in patients with relatively suboptimal nutritional parameters (albumin is <3 g/dl), we strongly consider a temporary, diverting, proximal jejunostomy for a period of 3–6 months with parenteral alimentation.

Prior to abdominal closure, the entire bowel surface should be inspected again very carefully to be certain that no unrecognized injuries exist. It is sometimes useful to check the adequacy of repair by inflating air (via syringe) into the bowel after filling the abdomen with saline to look for air leaks. Irrigation with a copious amount of warm saline is important. This practice increases the body temperature and corrects the associated coagulopathy after prolonged dissection and recovery from the anesthesia. We use closed suction drains in patients with no associated sepsis, whereas silastic passive drains are preferred in patients in the presence of residual sepsis. In patients with a prolonged operation and extensive dissection due to severe adhesions, we prefer to place a gastrostomy tube to avoid discomfort and the complications associated with a long-term nasogastric tube in the management of postoperative ileus. If possible, the omentum should be placed between the anastomosis and the incision.

Abdominal wall closure in patients with complex ECF can be challenging due to prior abdominal wall loss secondary to sepsis, evisceration, or herniation. Bowel wall edema with distention can also complicate the primary closure in these patients, especially with marked fluid administration. A primary abdominal closure is the preferred technique where possible. We avoid using permanent prosthetic material for abdominal closure, as this can lead to further fistulization. The primary aim in closing the abdomen of these patients is to bring the fascia and, whenever possible, the skin back together. Ventral hernias can be repaired later with synthetic mesh. The lateral release of the external oblique aponeurosis (components separation) can be helpful to allow primary fascia closure. If primary fascia closure is not possible, we use a technique of mobilizing full thickness skin flaps as lateral as possible, and close the skin tension-free with polypropylene suture in vertical mattress fashion over dental roles and staples to avoid any skin tear or necrosis (Figs. 7.3 and 7.4). When fascial approximation is not possible, it is important to lay the omentum or, or when no omentum is available, either a bioprosthesis like Alloderm or an absorbable polyglycolic acid mesh under this skin closure in case of wound breakdown; the omentum or the absorbable mesh can be covered with a skin graft or a vacuum-assisted dressing. We work with a plastic surgery team who has a special interest in and understanding of the pathophysiology of these complex cases; a musculocutaneous flap may be needed for primary closure or, in cases of direct exposure of the small bowel after the breakdown of the initial closure, a split-thickness skin graft. Skin grafting within lessthan 72h is important to avoid any further breakdown and fistulization of the small bowel.

The recovery of these patients can be difficult and prolonged. Active participation from a multidisciplinary team is imperative. The surgeon plays the primary role with assurance and emotional and mental support. Parenteral nutrition support in the postoperative period is essential and should be given until ileus resolves.

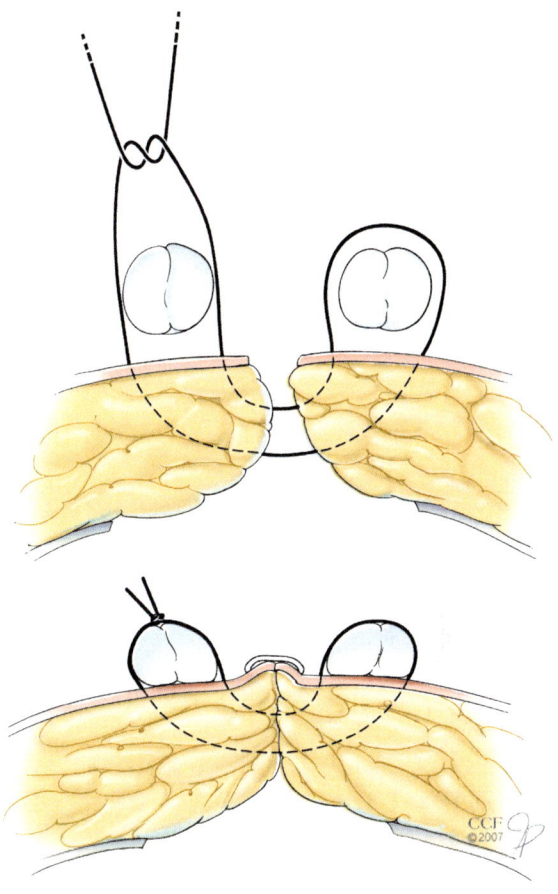

FIGURE 7.3. Abdominal wall closure at skin level with 1.0 polypropylene suture in vertical mattress over dental roles where primary fascia closure is not possible.

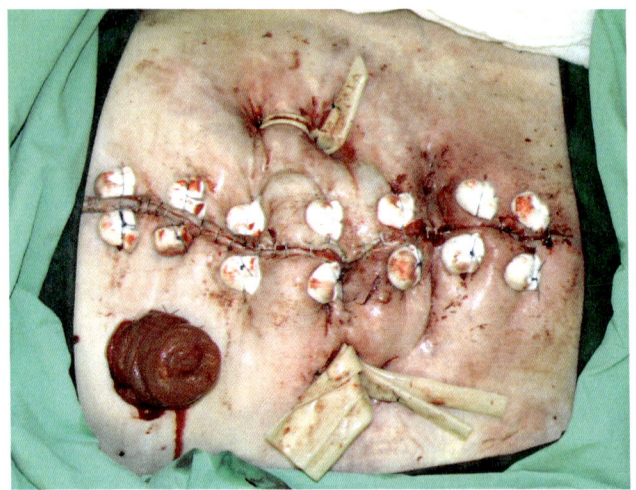

FIGURE 7.4. Complex wound closure where primary fascia closure is not possible.

Summary

The management of ECF is often a difficult problem. The principles of management involve control of sepsis and fistula output with adequate nutritional support. Early operative intervention in established ECF should be limited to abscess drainage and formation of a proximal defunctioning stoma for fistula effluent or sepsis control. The surgery of ECF is the surgery for adhesions, control of sepsis, and understanding the biology of this entire process – timing is everything. Definitive procedures for persistent ECF should be delayed to 4–6 months later with resection of the fistula and anastomosis of the healthy bowel. A low threshold is maintained for a defunctioning proximal stoma, particularly in the presence of residual sepsis, radiation enteritis, and Crohn's disease with multiple repair or resections. Operative and nonoperative management strategy, in the setting of a tertiary institution with access to multispecialty care, should result in a successful level of ECF closure with a low mortality and acceptable morbidity.

Selected Readings

Gibson SW, Fischer JE (2004) Enterocutaneous fistula. In: Fazio VW, Church JW, Delaney CP (eds) Current therapy in colon and rectal surgery. Mosby, St Louis, MO pp. 479–484

Gunn LA, Follmar KE, Wong MS et al. (2006) Management of enterocutaneous fistulas using negative pressure dressings. Ann Plast Surg 57:621–625

Lynch CA, Delaney CP, Senagore AJ et al. (2004) Clinical outcome and factors predictive of recurrence after enter-ocutaneous fistula surgery. Ann Surg 240:825–831

Makhdoom ZA, Komar MJ, Still CD (2003) Nutrition and enterocutaneous fistulas. J Clin Gastroenterol 31:195–204

Shetty V, Teubner A, Morrison K, Scott NA (2006) Proximal loop jejunostomy is a useful adjunct in the management of multiple intestinal suture lines in the septic abdomen. Brit J Surg 93:1247–1250

Worsey MJ, Fazio VW (2002) Reoperative pelvic surgery. In: Zuidema GD, Yeo CJ (eds) Shackelford's surgery of the alimentary tract, 5th edn, vol. 4. Elsevier, New York pp. 519–527

Part II
Malignant

8
Adenocarcinoma
of the Small Bowel

Shailesh V. Shrikhande and Supreeta Arya

Pearls and Pitfalls

- Malignant neoplasms of the small intestine are uncommon and account for less than 1% of all gastrointestinal (GI) tract neoplasms.
- Thirty-five percent to 50% of small bowel neoplasms are adenocarcinomas.
- Small bowel adenocarcinoma (SBA) is found in decreasing order of frequency in the duodenum, jejunum, and ileum.
- Geographic correlation between large and small bowel cancer suggests shared etiologies.
- Hereditary cancer syndromes, such as familial adenomatous polyposis (FAP), hereditary non-polyposis colorectal cancer (HNPCC), and Peutz-Jeghers syndrome (PJS), are all linked to development of SBA.
- Crohn's disease is associated with an increased risk of SBA with a risk approximately 12-fold greater than the general population.
- Remember to consider a small bowel neoplasm when patients present with non-specific abdominal complaints or unexplained anemia.
- SBA is detected earlier than other small intestinal cancers. In particular, adenocarcinomas of the ampulla and the duodenum manifest earlier than SBA elsewhere in the jejunum and ileum. Thus, SBA in this region results in obstructive jaundice which aids in a somewhat earlier detection.

K.I. Bland et al. (eds.), *Surgery of the Small Bowel*,
DOI: 10.1007/978-1-84996-372-5_8,
© Springer-Verlag London Limited 2011

- Diagnostic tests to be used include upper gastrointestinal endoscopy, colonoscopy, computed tomography, and lastly a small bowel study to visualize the small bowel, especially if the upper and lower gastrointestinal studies are negative. Double contrast small bowel examination, or enteroclysis, is currently the best technique that can be employed for accurate information regarding the status of the small intestine.
- Operative resection is the treatment of choice and the only therapeutic modality with a curative potential.
- Pancreatoduodenectomy and local ampullary excision are the two available options for duodenal/ ampullary disease.
- Local resection of periampullary neoplasms has a high rate of recurrence (5–30%) and requires an aggressive long-term postoperative endoscopic surveillance.
- Small bowel resection with wide surgical margins is the treatment for SBA located in the duodenum as well as in the jejunum and ileum.
- Distal ileal lesions may necessitate a right hemicolectomy.
- Five-year survival after resection is approximately 30% with a median survival of 20 months.
- Adjuvant treatment has no definite role in SBA except possibly in periampullary adenocarcinoma.

Introduction

The length of the small intestine is approximately 5 to 7 m and constitutes 60% of the gastrointestinal (GI) tract. Despite its length and an exposure to a wide spectrum of carcinogens, malignant neoplasms of the small intestine are uncommon and account for less than 1% of all GI tract neoplasms. The age-adjusted incidence of small bowel malignancies is 1/100,000 with a prevalence of 0.6%. Compared with other GI neoplasms, information about small intestinal malignant neoplasms is rather limited, and this is not surprising given that estimated malignant neoplasms of the small intestine are 40–70 times less common than colonic carcinoma. Despite the fact that the small intestine represents 90% of the absorptive surface of the GI tract, the average, annual, age-adjusted incidence of small bowel cancer is 50 times less common than colorectal cancer in the United States. While 35–50% of small bowel neoplasms are adenocarcinomas, 20–40% are carcinoids, 5–14% are lymphomas, and 15% are sarcomas (i.e. Gastrointestinal Stromal Tumors, or GIST). Small bowel adenocarcinoma accounts for 2% of GI neoplasms and 1% of GI cancer deaths.

The sites at highest risk of developing malignant neoplasms are the duodenum for adenocarcinoma and the ileum for carcinoids and lymphomas. Small bowel adenocarcinoma (SBA) is found in decreasing order of frequency in the duodenum, jejunum, and ileum. Recently, incidence data from the Surveillance, Epidemiology, and End Results (SEER) program (1973–2000) were used to analyze the four histologic types of small bowel cancer, viz., adenocarcinomas, carcinoid neoplasms, lymphomas, and sarcomas. This study observed that men had higher rates than women for all types of small bowel cancer. African-Americans had almost double the incidence of carcinomas and carcinoid neoplasms compared to Caucasians (10.6 vs. 5.6 per million people; 9.2 vs. 5.4 per million people, respectively). Furthermore, the geographic correlation between large and small bowel cancer suggested shared etiologies.

Risk Factors and Pathogenesis

In a study evaluating risk factors for SBA, the intake of bread, pasta, or rice appeared to increase directly the risk of small bowel cancer. In contrast, risk correlated inversely with coffee, fish, vegetables, and fruit. These results seem to suggest that dietary correlates of SBA are similar to those of colon cancer and at least of the same magnitude. While this particular study failed to confirm a definite association between smoking and alcohol consumption and development of small bowel cancer, other studies have shown that such a relationship exists. Epithelial cells of the GI tract are often exposed to toxic agents such as 7, 12-dimethylbenzanthracene (DMBA), the phenothiazines, and benzpyrene.

Clinical Conditions Predisposing to Increased Risk of SBA

A number of clinical conditions are known to increase the risk of SBA. Hereditary cancer syndromes, such as familial adenomatous polyposis (FAP), hereditary non-polyposis colorectal cancer (HNPCC), and Peutz-Jeghers syndrome (PJS), are all linked to development of SBA. The lifetime risk of developing an HNPCC-related SBA is estimated to range 1–4%, which is 100 times greater than in the general population. Compared to the general population, SBA in the setting of HNPCC presents at an earlier age and carries a better prognosis compared to sporadic SBA. For PJS, a meta-analysis revealed a greater risk of gastrointestinal cancer and more specifically for SBA associated with PJS. There is evidence to suggest that PJS-related cancers have different underlying molecular genetic alterations compared with SBA that arise in the sporadic setting. Duodenal adenomas which are usually located around the ampulla of Vater for unknown reasons occur in 31–92% patients of FAP. Endoscopic examination at periodic intervals may be worthwhile to screen for early neoplasms in these FAP patients. Crohn's disease is also associated with an increased risk of SBA of 12-fold greater than the general population. In Crohn's disease, the small bowel neoplasms appear at a younger age compared to sporadic SBA and tend to be more common in the distal part of the small intestine where the Crohn's disease is usually active. Most SBAs associated with Crohn's disease are localized within an inflammatory stricture, where they are often responsible for obstructive disease. Risk factors for SBA in patients of Crohn's disease include male sex, previous surgical bypass loops, chronic fistulous disease, and long-standing disease of at least 10 years. Celiac disease has also been linked to development of SBA; however, its etiology remains uncertain. A distinctive feature of celiac disease-associated SBA is that the neoplasms tend to be localized in the jejunum and are often lymphomas. The various clinical conditions predisposing to SBA are listed in Table 8.1.

TABLE 8.1. Clinical conditions predisposing to increased risk of small bowel cancer.

Hereditary non-polyposis colorectal cancer syndrome (HNPCC)

Peutz-Jegher syndrome (PJS)

Familial adenomatous polyposis syndrome (FAP)

Crohn's disease

Celiac disease

Neurofibromatosis type I (NF-I)

Molecular Genetics of SBA

The adenoma-carcinoma sequence in colorectal cancer represents a series of well-defined molecular changes consisting of activation of oncogenes and inactivation of tumor suppressor genes that accompany the histologic progression to invasive cancer. While similarities between small bowel and large bowel cancer suggest that they share many of the molecular changes of carcinogenesis, clear evidence is either lacking or limited. In a recent study evaluating the genetic pathway of SBA, Wheeler and colleagues investigated the expression of mismatch repair genes hMLH1 and hMSH2, the adenomatous polyposis coli (APC) gene, β–catenin, E-cadherin, and p53 in SBA. They did not observe any mutations in the mutation cluster region (MCR) of the APC gene, which suggests that adenocarcinoma of the small intestine may follow a somewhat different genetic pathway to colorectal cancer. Furthermore, abnormal expression of b-catenin and E-cadherin suggested an early pathway in which mutations could be found in SBA. Overexpression of p53 is a frequent finding. Similar to colorectal cancer, this event reflects its important role in carcinogenesis in the small intestine. A number of studies have detected K-ras mutations in 14–83% of cases of SBA; however, this difference was reported over a wide range, because the number of duodenal adenocarcinomata within these studies were often of a small sample size. Some authors demonstrated complete concordance in K-ras mutations between

TABLE 8.2. Possible reasons for rarity of small bowel adenocarcinoma compared to colorectal cancers.

Shorter bowel transit time with reduced exposure between mucosa and carcinogens

Large volume of secretions dilute insult of carcinogens on mucosa

Bacterial degradation of bile salts does not occur in small intestine

Lower level of anerobes in small intestine

Presence of abundant lymphoid tissue

Rapid proliferation of small bowel cells causes competitive inhibition of malignant cells at tumor site

tissues from adenocarcinomas and contiguous adenomas in their case series. This observation suggests a relationship between the conventional adenoma-carcinoma sequence and K-ras mutation in small bowel cancer. The oncogene c-neu is altered in approximately 50% of sporadic colorectal cancer cases; in SBA, 60% of these neoplasms were positive for this mutation. Furthermore, oncogene expression was noted to increase directly with tumor grade. Patients with c-neu positive neoplasms had a shorter survival compared to those with c-neu negative neoplasms. The potential reasons for the rarity of small bowel adenocarcinoma compared to colorectal cancer are provided in Table 8.2.

Clinical Presentation and Diagnosis

Unfortunately, small bowel tumors and cancers usually do not manifest with definite classic symptoms. Therefore, it is important to consider a small bowel tumor when patients present with non-specific abdominal complaints or unexplained anemia. The usual diagnostic tests used in the presence of such complaints are upper gastrointestinal endoscopy, colonoscopy, and lastly small bowel radiography to visualize the small bowel, especially if the upper and lower gastrointestinal studies are negative. Another symptom which an alert clinician could suspect and diagnose a small bowel tumor is that of insidious bowel obstruction – colicky abdominal pain and a sensation of abdominal distension. A plain x-ray of the abdomen during such episodes of "non-specific" abdominal complaints may reveal air fluid levels and point to a small bowel obstruction. Such a finding, however, indicates that the disease has progressed beyond the "early stage" of small bowel cancer. In early stage or asymptomatic small bowel cancers, plain x-rays of the abdomen have their limitations as does the barium meal follow-through which is widely available, simple, and inexpensive, but insensitive for detection of small or early SBA. Instead, double-contrast small bowel examination or enteroclysis is the best technique currently that can be employed for accurate information regarding the status of the small intestine. Barium and methylcellulose are infused in the small bowel under pressure which produces distension of the small bowel, thereby enabling the radiologist to follow the contrast material throughout its course in the small intestine. Furthermore, this examination offers the advantage of evaluating the mucosa for irregularities; hence this method is the best technique that is available widely and relatively inexpensive. Computerized tomography-aided enteroclysis, combining CT with enteroclysis, is considered an even better diagnostic test in small bowel cancers (Fig. 8.1). The ability to image accurately a small intestinal neoplasm, independent of its size, anatomic localization, and growth characteristics, represents a major improvement in the diagnosis and management of small bowel cancer (Fig. 8.2). The most recent investigational development has been the introduction of capsule endoscopy in addition to push enteroscopy, Sonde enteroscopy, and intraoperative or laparoscopically assisted enteroscopy. Capsule endoscopy consists of a video capsule that is swallowed and transmits images from the small intestine. The major limitation with this technique is the lack of external control over the position and orientation of the capsule and the high cost of this technology. Push enteroscopy enables examination of the jejunum for 40–60 cm distal to the ligament of Treitz with the help of a longer endoscope.

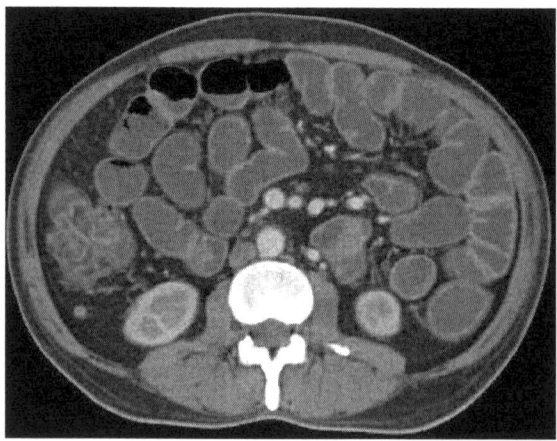

FIGURE 8.1. Axial section of CT enteroclysis showing water distended normal small bowel loops with thin smooth walls.

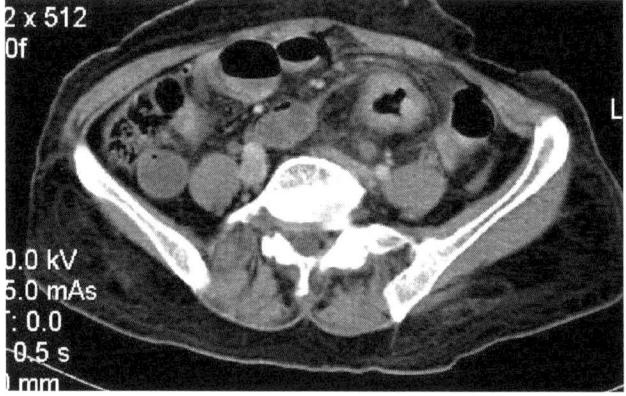

FIGURE 8.2. Axial contrast enhanced CT showing concentric wall thickening in a short segment of small bowel (ileum) confirmed histologically to be adenocarcinoma (From the Archives of Department of Radiology, KEM Hospital, Mumbai, India. Courtesy of Professor Ravi Ramakantan).

Intraoperative endoscopy is a variant of push enteroscopy in which the surgeon can guide the endoscope inserted per orally or a colonoscope passed per rectum. Intraoperative endoscopy should, however, be the last resort for the clinician in suspected early stage small bowel cancer, because it is a major invasive procedure involving laparotomy.

In duodenal and ampullary adenocarcinoma, the presentation is somewhat different, and usually with signs and symptoms of upper abdominal pain, gastric outlet obstruction, and jaundice.

Treatment of SBA

SBA is detected earlier than other small intestinal cancers. In particular, adenocarcinomas of the ampulla and the duodenum manifest earlier than SBA elsewhere in the jejunum and ileum. Thus, SBA in this region results in obstructive jaundice which occasionally aids in a somewhat earlier detection. Despite this observation, the majority of SBA are metastatic at the time of diagnosis.

Surgical Treatment of SBA

Duodenal and Ampullary Adenocarcinoma

Operative resection is the treatment of choice and the only therapeutic modality with a curative potential. Pancreatoduodenectomy and local ampullary excision are the two available options. Local resection has a high rate of recurrence (5–30%) and requires postoperative endoscopic surveillance, which is the reason it is not considered as a first choice in the management of ampullary neoplasms. In a study evaluating 92 patients with cancer of the ampulla of Vater, 10 were treated with local resection, 49 with pancreatic resection, and 33 underwent only a laparotomy without resection. When the main outcome measures of postoperative morbidity and mortality, surgical radicality, and long-term survival were evaluated, the postoperative complication rate was significantly less after local resection, whereas mortality did not differ between the two operated groups. UICC stages were significantly less advanced in the local resection group; also, the frequency of positive resection margins and R0 resections was the same in both groups, as was long-term survival. The local recurrence rate, however, was 80% after local resection and 22% after pancreatic resection. The conclusion was that pancreatoduodenectomy should be the preferred operation for cancer of the ampulla of Vater in patients who are fit for major surgery, whereas local resection may be considered in carefully selected patients. A number of other earlier studies have also reached similar conclusions.

Because local resection is less invasive, it has been argued that it is potentially an equally effective alternative for cancers with favorable prognostic features. Thus, identification of these prognostic parameters may allow selection of some patients suitable for local resection. In a study evaluating 25 patients with primary adenocarcinoma of ampulla treated by pancreatoduodenectomy and local resection, it was observed that T-staging could predict the risk of tumor recurrence and could be determined accurately using endoscopic ultrasonography. Local resection was concluded to be a suitable alternative to pancreatoduodenal resection in patients with T1-and T2-adenocarcinomas with a maximum diameter of 3 cm or less. A word of caution about local ampullary resection is required. This procedure can be demanding and requires skill and understanding of the local anatomy; it is inadvisable for an inexperienced general surgeon to proceed with this operation without advice from an experienced biliary-pancreatic surgeon.

In summary, with an operative mortality of 5% or less for pancreatoduodenectomy, it is currently the procedure of choice at most experienced centers for invasive carcinoma, foci of papillary adenocarcinoma in pre-excisional biopsies, or in ampullary adenomas with high-grade dysplasia. Ampullectomy is reserved for benign adenomas. It must be acknowledged that pancreatoduodenectomy is curative in 80% of patients with node-negative ampullary carcinomas; once 3-year survival is reached, long-term survival can be expected. The choice of treatment, however, depends on the level of surgical skill available, availability of endoscopic ultrasonography, and local expertise, patient compliance, and the presence or absence of co-existing familial adenomatous polyposis. Non-ampullary duodenal adenomas (FAP) can also be treated by a pancreas-preserving duodenectomy. An experienced biliopancreatic surgeon is crucial to ensure safe outcomes with use of this uncommon procedure.

Table 8.3 lists the outcomes of major series ampullary and duodenal adenocarcinoma treated by pancreatoduodenectomy.

TABLE 8.3. Major series of outcomes after treatment of ampullary and duodenal adenocarcinoma with pancreatoduodenectomy.

Tumor location	Author	5-year survival
Ampulla (overall)	De Castro SM et al., 2004	37%
Ampulla (overall)	Di Giorgio et al., 2005	64.40%
Ampulla (overall)	Roberts RH et al., 1999	46%
Ampulla (node negative)	Brown et al., 2005	78%
Ampulla (T1 and T2 lesions)	Brown et al., 2005	73%
Ampulla (well differentiated)	Brown et al., 2005	76%
Ampulla (node positive)	Brown et al., 2005	25%
Ampulla (T3 and T4 tumors)	Brown et al., 2005	8%
Ampulla (moderately/ poorly differentiated)	Brown et al., 2005	36%
Duodenal	Schmidt et al., 2004	42% (3-year survival)
Ampulla		53% (3-year survival)
Duodenal	Sun et al., 2004	45.40%
Duodenal	Bakaeen et al., 2000	54%
Duodenal	Sohn et al., 1998	53%

The various prognostic factors influencing survival in duodenal and ampullary adenocarcinoma are provided in Table 8.4. Patients with unresectable lesions should be treated symptomatically. Biliary obstruction and jaundice should be treated by endoscopic stenting (plastic/metallic stenting), while gastroduodenal obstruction is treated by palliative surgical gastric bypass.

Jejunal and Ileal Adenocarcinoma

These lesions are treated by radical, segmental small bowel resection en bloc with the mesentery and its lymphatic drainage. Adequate proximal and distal pathologically negative margins must be ensured. Equally good results are achieved by both hand-sewn and stapler anastomoses. Terminal ileal lesions may have to treated by right hemicolectomy.

Management of Advanced Disease

Management of this state offers special challenges especially for those who are not eligible for palliative surgery. Treatment revolves around nasogastric aspiration, intravenous fluids, total parenteral nutrition, and in some cases antispasmodic agents.

TABLE 8.4. Prognostic factors influencing survival in duodenal and ampullary adenocarcinoma.

Lymph node positivity
Type of surgery (pancreatoduodenectomy vs. local resection)
Experience of the treating center in major resectional surgery
(<16 pancreatoduodenectomies/year)
Patient age (>75 years)
Patient reluctance for major definitive surgery (>75 years)

Adjuvant Treatment for SBA

The leading cause of death from SBA is distant metastatic disease. This observation suggests that adjuvant chemotherapy should have a role in management of SBA. Unfortunately, no chemotherapy in use is of proven benefit, although many periampullary adenocarcinomas may be given adjuvant therapy with an occasional excellent result.

Conclusion

Early diagnosis is crucial for the definitive treatment of SBA. Oncologic surgery provides superior outcomes, thus, referral to specialist centers is to be preferred. According to a landmark study by the American College of Surgeons Commission on Cancer, the overall 5-year disease-specific survival of 5000 SBAs was 31% with a median survival of 20 months. Adjuvant chemotherapy is of unproven benefit in all SBA.

Selected Readings

Bakaeen FG, Murr MM, Sarr MG, Thompson GB, Farnell MB, Nagorney DM, Farley DR, van Heerden JA, Wiersema LM, Schleck CD, Donohue JH (2000). What prognostic factors are important in duodenal adenocarcinoma? Arch Surg. 135(6):635–641; discussion 641–2

Brown KM, Tompkins AJ, Yong S et al. (2005) Pancreaticoduodenectomy is curative in the majority of patients with node-negative ampullary cancer. Arch Surg 140:529–532; discussion 532–533

de Castro SM, van Heek NT, Kuhlmann KF et al. (2004) Surgical management of neoplasms of the ampulla of Vater: local resection or pancreatoduodenectomy and prognostic factors for survival. Surgery 136:994–1002

Delaunoit T, Neczyporenko F, Limburg PJ, Erlichman C (2005) Pathogenesis and risk factors of small bowel adeno-carcinoma: a colorectal cancer sibling? Am J Gastroenterol 100:703–710

Di Giorgio A, Alfieri S, Rotondi F et al. (2005) Pancreato-duodenectomy for tumors of Vater's ampulla: report on 94 consecutive patients. World J Surg 29:513–518

120   S.V. Shrikhande and S. Arya

Frost DB, Mercado PD, Tyrell JS (1994) Small bowel cancer: a 30-year review. Ann Surg Oncol 1:290–295

Haselkorn T, Whittemore AS, Lilienfeld DE (2005) Incidence of small bowel cancer in the United States and worldwide: geographic, temporal, and racial differences. Cancer Causes Control 16:781–787

Howe JR, Karnell LH, Menck HR, Scott-Conner C (1999) The American College of Surgeons Commission on Cancer and the American Cancer Society. Adenocarcinoma of the small bowel: review of the National Cancer Data Base, 1985–1995. Cancer 86:2693–706

Jones DV, Skibber J, Levin B (1998) Adenocarcinoma and other small intestinal neoplasms, including benign tumors. In: Feldman M, Scharschmidt BF (eds) Sleisenger gastro-intestinal and liver disease. W.B. Saunders, Philadelphia, pp. 1858–1865

Lewis JD, Deren JJ, Lichtenstein GR (1999) Cancer risk in patients with inflammatory bowel disease. Gastroenterol Clin North Am 28:459–77

Lynch HT, Smyrk TC, Lynch PM et al. (1989) Adenocarcinoma of the small bowel in lynch syndrome II. Cancer 64:2178–2183

Roberts RH, Krige JE, Bornman PC, Terblanche J (1999). Pancreatic-oduodenectomy of ampullary carcinoma. Am Surg. 65(11):1043–1048

Schmidt CM, Powell ES, Yiannoutsos CT et al. (2004) Pancreaticoduodenectomy: a 20-year experience in 516 patients. Arch Surg 139: 718–275; discussion 725–727

Sohn TA, Lillemoe KD, Cameron JL, Pitt HA, Kaufman HS, Hruban RH, Yeo CJ (1998). Adenocarcinoma of the duodenum: factors influencing long-term survival. J Gastrointest Surg. 2(1):79–87

Sun JJ, Wu ZY (2004). Treatment of 54 cases of primary malignant duodenal tumor. Zhonghua Wai Ke Za Zhi., 42(5):276–278

Talamonti MS, Goetz LH, Rao S, Joehl RJ (2002) Primary cancers of the small bowel: analysis of prognostic factors and results of surgical management. Arch Surg 137:564–570; discussion 570–571

Vasen HF, Wijnen JT, Menko FH et al. (1996) Cancer risk in families with hereditary nonpolyposis colorectal cancer diagnosed by mutation analysis. Gastroenterology 110:1020–1027

Wheeler JM, Warren BF, Mortensen NJ et al. (2002) An insight into the genetic pathway of adenocarcinoma of the small intestine. Gut 50:218–223

Younes N, Fulton N, Tanaka R et al. (1997) The presence of K-12 ras mutations in duodenal adenocarcinomas and the absence of ras mutations in other small bowel adeno-carcinomas and carcinoid tumors. Cancer 79:1804–1808

9
Lymphoma of the Small Bowel

Wing-Yan Au and Raymond H.S. Liang

Pearls and Pitfalls

- Lymphoma of the small bowel present with local gastrointestinal or systemic symptoms, including malabsorption, mass lesions, bowel obstruction, bleeding, and/or systemic symptoms.
- The most common histology is diffuse large B-cell lymphoma, but mucosa-associated lymphoid tissue lymphoma (MALToma), mantle cell lymphoma, and mature T-cell lymphoma can occur.
- Surgical de-bulking is often required due to the size and complications caused by the lesions. An R0 resection may not be crucial, but lymphoma involvement of an anastomosis should be avoided for concern of leakage during chemotherapy.
- Lymphoma is a systemic disease, and systemic chemotherapy is needed, even for localized lesions with complete resection. For small or apparently unresectable lesions, biopsy followed by chemotherapy is preferred to extensive resection.
- An adequate wedge-type (not FNA) biopsy is necessary for histologic diagnosis, classification, and appropriate treatment. Specific treatment may be needed for different

K.I. Bland et al. (eds.), *Surgery of the Small Bowel*,
DOI: 10.1007/978-1-84996-372-5_9,
© Springer-Verlag London Limited 2011

lineage and various histologic subtypes of lymphoma; thus, proper handling of the specimen is needed. Sending fresh tissue to the pathology laboratory is desirable for proper immuno-staining and molecular lineage clarification.
• Prognosis varies widely, depending on histology and stage.

Introduction

Lymphoma of the small bowel constitutes 2% of all extra-nodal lymphomas. Small bowel lymphoma, including ileocecal and multiple sites of involvement, accounts for about 20% of all small bowel malignancies and about 25% of all gastrointestinal lymphomas. Small bowel is the second most common site of lymphoma gut involvement, after the stomach. Primary intestinal lymphoma arises from lymphoid cells present in the Peyer's patches. The incidence of lymphoma decreases from the ileum to jejunum to duodenum. Lymphoma is a heterogeneous disease in terms of biology and clinical behavior due to the great variety of normal lymphocytes. The World Health Organization (WHO) classification divides lymphoma biologically into B-and T-/ natural killer (NK) cell lineages (Table 9.1). The incidence of the various subtypes varies widely; some lesions appear to be peculiar to particular sites and ethnic groups. The common subtypes of lymphoma that occur in the gastrointestinal tract are highlighted below.

Clinical Presentation

Most series report a peak presentation in the 7th decade with a 2:1 male predominance. Due to the inaccessibility of the small bowel to clinical examination, and endoscopic and radiologic imaging, the diagnosis of small bowel lymphoma may be difficult and is often delayed. Local symptoms are similar to those caused by other malignant or non-malignant intestinal lesions, including pain (85%), mass bowel obstruction due to intussusception (26%), bleeding (22%), and rupture (23%). For rapidly growing lesions, such as Burkitt's

TABLE 9.1. World Health Organization classification of lymphomas with the four main categories of B-cell, T-/NK-cell/Hodgkin/and immunodeficiency-related lymphomas.

Mature B cell neoplasms	Mature T/NK neoplasms	Immunodeficiency lymphoma
*Diffuse large cell lymphoma	Peripheral T cell NOS	HIV related
*Extranodal marginal zone (MALToma)	*T/ NK nasal/ nasal type	Post transplant lymphoma
Follicular lymphoma	*Enteropathic T cell	Primary/secondary immune disorders
*Mantle cell lymphoma		
*Burkitt lymphoma		
Lymphoplasmacytoid/ Waldenstrom	Anaplastic large cell	
Plasma cell neoplasms	Hepatosplenic T cell	Hodgkin's lymphoma
B-Prolymphocytic leukemia	Mycosis fungoides	Nodular lymphocyte predominant
Chronic lymphocytic leukemia/SLL	Primary cutaneous CD30 T cell	Lymphocyte rich classical
Hairy cell leukemia	Subcutaneous panniculitis	Classical
	T-large granular lymphocytosis	Nodular sclerosis classical
	T-prolymphocytic leukemia	Mixed cellularity

*Entities encountered in the small bowel.

lymphoma and NK lymphoma, local symptoms can be dramatic. Lymphoma of the small bowel is a great mimicker of conditions, including tuberculosis and Crohn's disease, and may cause unexplained systemic features such as fever and weight loss (in one-third of patients), while defying extensive investigations. Late presentation is not unusual. An increased serum lactate dehydrogenase level (LDH) may be a clue. The use of PET (Fig. 9.1) may be useful for localization of the

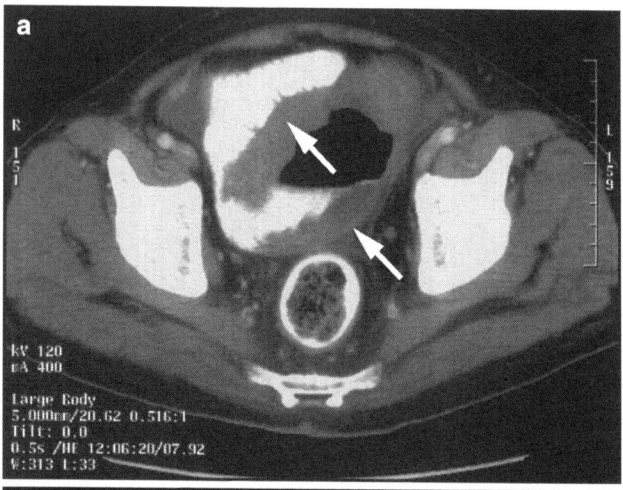

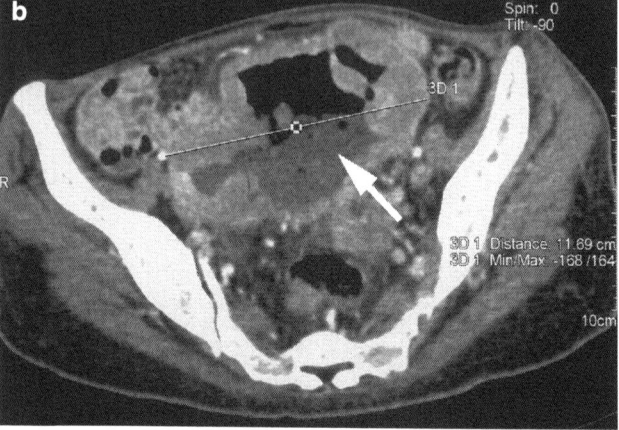

FIGURE 9.1. CT and PET-CT images of the four different presentations of small bowel lymphoma. (**a**) Multiple segments of bowel wall thickening in a patient with anemia. (**b**) Acute perforation of the small bowel walled off by omentum resulting in an intra-abdominal abscess. (**c**) Patient had a history of systemic lupus erythematosus on prolonged azathioprine. PET scan showed single focus of tumor in small bowel. Resection revealed Epstein Barr virus-positive immunosuppression-related lymphoma. (**d**) Huge intra-abdominal mass in a patient with rapidly growing Burkitt's lymphoma.

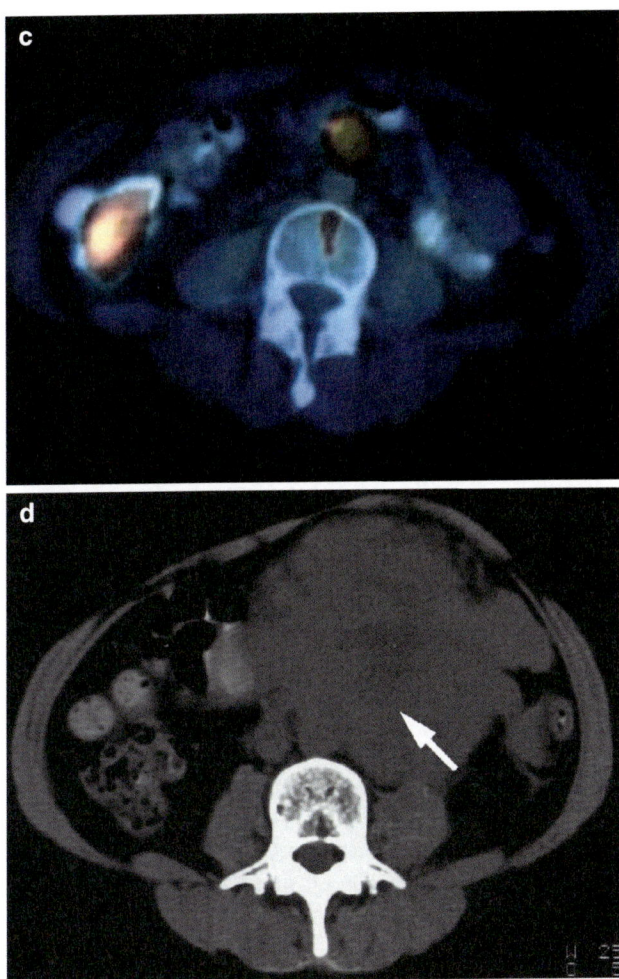

FIGURE 9.1. (continued).

disease. Certain subgroups of patients are at increased risk for specific small bowel lymphoma, including patients with celiac disease, those on immunosuppression due to transplantation, HIV infection, or congenital immunodeficiency, patients with nodular lymphoid hyperplasia of the intestine,

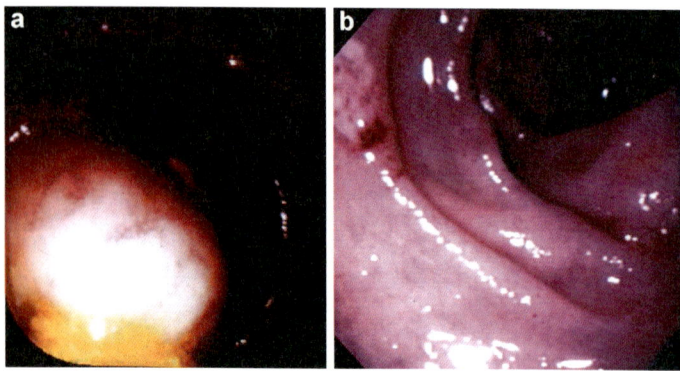

FIGURE 9.2. Endoscopic appearances. Two B-cell lymphomas involving parts of small bowel accessible by endoscopy (biopsies confirmed small bowel lymphoma). (**a**) MALToma appearing as a duodenal polyp. (**b**) Thickening of ileocecal fold by mantle cell lymphoma on multiple biopsies.

and those of Middle Eastern descent. Due to the mucosa homing nature of small bowel lymphocytes, multiple sites of small bowel may be involved by lymphoma (10%) (Fig. 9.2).

Pathology and Classification

According to Lee et al., two-thirds of the primary lymphomas of small intestine are of B-cell lineage, and 60–80% of both B-and T-cell small bowel lymphoma are classified as high-grade lesions (Lee et al., 2004). In most clinical and pathological series, gastrointestinal lymphomas are discussed as one single entity (Liang et al). However, in both etiological and clinical terms, the spectrum of origin and behavior of small bowel lymphoma are vastly different from that of gastric lymphoma. The prognosis and optimal treatment for each WHO category are also different and these clinical series are difficult to interpret without the pathological details.

Diffuse large B-cell lymphoma: Similar to lymphomas of nodal origin, diffuse B-cell histology accounts for 50% of all small bowel lymphomas. Unlike those in the stomach, transformation from MALToma (Lymphoma of mucosa-associated lymphoid tissue) is uncommon. Regional lymph node involvement and systemic involvement occurs in 10–15% of patients. Histologically, sheets of large centroblasts or immunoblasts do not usually form follicular structure (Fig. 9.3a). The cells are usually positive for CD20 and bcl-6, signifying a germinal center origin. The response to chemotherapy is good even though relapse, often extraintestinal, may occur in 30% of patients.

Low-grade lymphomas: MALTomas arise from the mucosa-associated lymphoid tissue in the submucosal region. Concomitant lymphoma may be present in the stomach, large bowel, and other mucosal areas, such as eye, lung, and salivary glands. Histologically, the malignant lymphoid cells are small in size and show distinct lympho-epithelial lesions (Fig. 9.3b) and glandular destruction. The cells are positive for CD20 but negative for CD5, CD10 and bcl-6. Secondary transformation to large cells and diffuse histology may occur. The behavior is indolent, but eradication of gastric Helicobacter pylori may cause regression of the gastric forms. Both follicular lymphoma, as well as small cell lymphoma, may have primary and isolated small intestinal presentation. The prognosis is good, and their relation to the more common nodal and disseminated disease is undefined.

Mantle cell lymphoma: This is an aggressive lymphoma that arises from the mantle zone of the lymphoid follicle. Although a systemic disease, the malignant mantle cells home to the intestine and up to 70% of patients have small and large intestinal involvement at autopsy (lymphomatous polyposis). The growth is monotonous and cells are positive for CD5, CD20, and bcl-1. The disease usually runs a relentless, fatal, relapsing course.

Burkitt's lymphoma: This is a rare, but alarmingly rapid-growing progressive neoplasm. Classically occurring in a cervical, ovary, and neck node, it is also common in the small bowel. A classic "starry sky" appearance is evident on histology due to extensive cell apoptosis and mitoses. The cells express CD20 and Ki-67 and are also positive for Epstein Barr virus (EBV) in patients with HIV. Response to

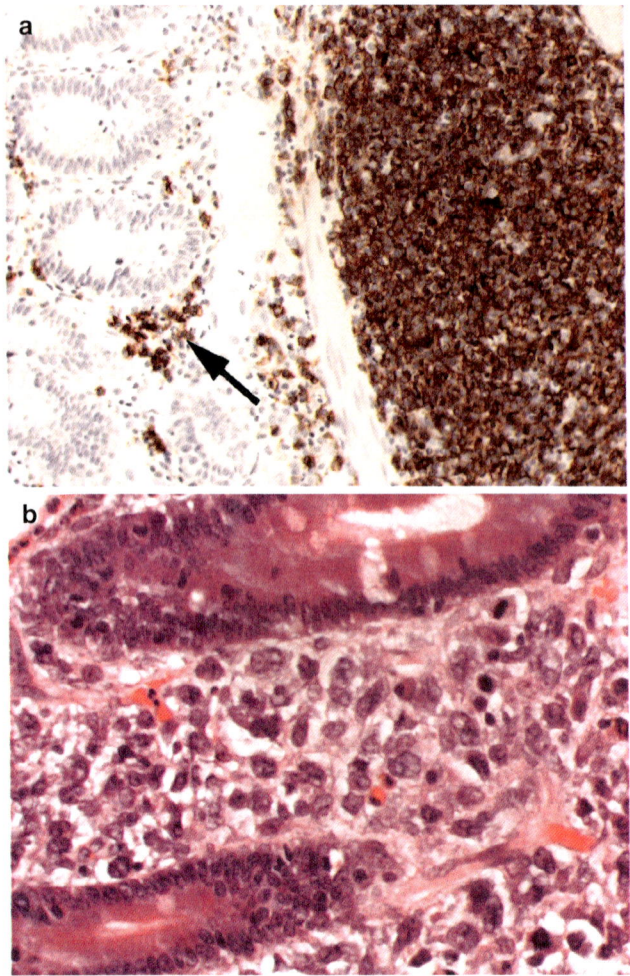

FIGURE 9.3. (**a**) Mucosal and submucosal infiltration by sheets of CD20-positive, diffuse large B cell lymphoma, stained brown by immunohistochemistry. There is no evidence of invasion of the mucosal villi (*arrow*). (**b**) Hematoxylin and eosin staining showing diffuse large B cell lymphoma on high power. (**c**) An NK cell lymphoma of small bowel presenting as perforation with sheets of lymphoma cells with necrosis. (**d**) High power view showing angioinvasion by malignant NK cells (*arrow*) (Histologic appearances courtesy of Dr. Tony W. H. Shek, Queen Mary Hospital, Hong Kong).

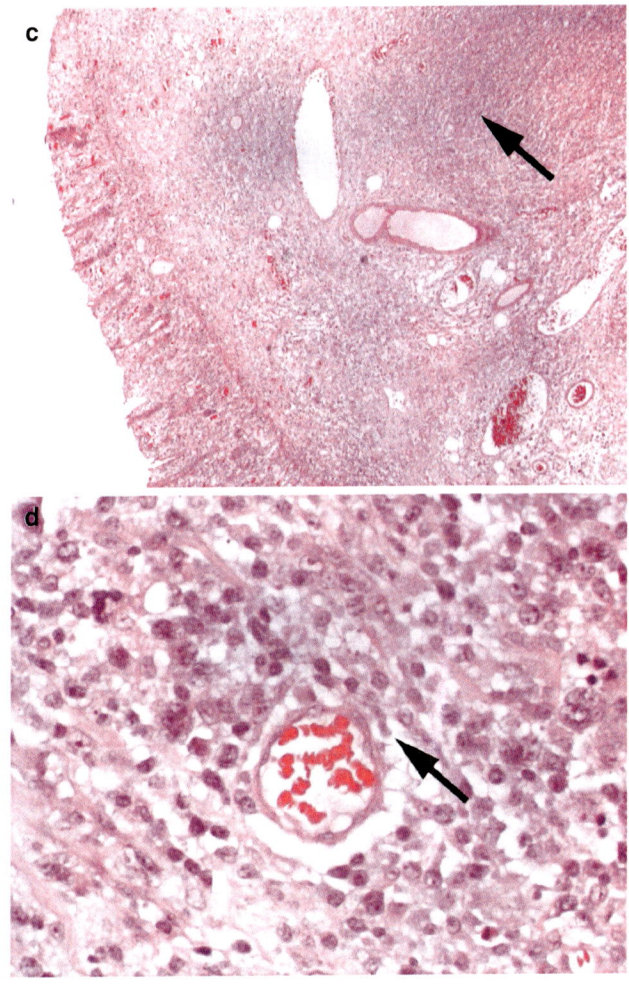

FIGURE 9.3. (continued).

chemotherapy is rapid, and the whole lesion may disappear within hours. Despite such a rapid response, however, prognosis is poor with relapses occurring systemically and in the central nervous system. Aggressive treatment with hemopoietic stem cell transplantation may be required.

Lymphoplasmacytoid lymphoma: This is an indolent zlymphoma that secretes monoclonal immunoglobulins (alpha chain disease). It is more commonly seen in certain ethnic groups, e.g., in patients of Middle Eastern descent (immunoproliferative small intestinal disease or IPSID) and is associated with bacterial overgrowth and malabsorption. Campylobacter jejuni has been implicated as the antigenic stimuli in some patients. The lymphoid cells show a classic plasmacytic differentiation. Chemotherapy and antibiotic treatment usually provide good disease control. Despite aggressive treatment, prognosis is poor for the transformed cases.

Mature T-cell lymphoma: This mixed group of disease constitutes 15–30% of all small bowel lymphomas, depending on the different ethnic groups and geographic areas. In Asian countries, peripheral T-cell lymphoma and NK-/T and EBV-positive nasal-type lymphoma predominate. The lymphoid cells are medium in size, positive for CD3E, and negative for B-cell markers. EBV association is common for PTCL and invariable for NK lymphoma. The latter are also CD56 positive, accounting for its intestinal preference due to homotypic attraction. Due to its aggressive growth, bowel perforation is common, and the prognosis is poor. In Caucasians, enteropathic T-cell lymphoma may follow expansion of intraepithelial T-cells, resulting in celiac disease and refractory sprue. Gluten-free diet may reduce the risk. Prognosis is usually dismal due to its late diagnosis and malnutrition.

Imaging and Endoscopic Appearance

The small intestine is a difficult part of the body for imaging despite the use of intravenous, oral, and air contrast techniques of imaging. The diagnostic sensitivities of contrast radiography, computed tomography, and endoscopic biopsy are all reported to be over 75%, but up to 10–25% of small bowel lymphoma may only be detectable at operation, especially for the diffuse types. For lymphoma forming mass lesions (30%), mesenteric and retroperitoneal lymphadenopathy (50%), and bowel wall

thickening (70%), CT is preferred over MRI. Most lymphomas are contrast-enhancing and homogeneous in attenuation,
but large lesions may have areas of necrosis. In most cases, it
is impossible to differentiate lymphoma from other neoplasms
by imaging. The use of CT-guided core biopsy may obviate the
need for open laparotomy for some bulky lesions. Although
gallium scintigraphy may pick up lymphomatous lesions, its
sensitivity in the small bowel is low. PET scanning is useful
in high-risk patients and simplifies localization and staging.
But PET scan may be negative for low-grade lymphomas, e.g.,
MALToma. The use of virtual endoscopy (MRI or CT) has not
been evaluated. Because staging is an integral part of management, full staging by CT/MRI/PET screening of the thorax,
abdomen, and pelvis is necessary.

The ability to perform endoscopic biopsy, coupled with
imaging, may avoid the need for open laparotomy in treating
some small bowel lymphomas, although concomitant involvement of the gastric and colonic regions, the regions most amenable to endoscopic access, is usually not be present. In
addition, lymphoma usually does not extend to the parts of
the duodenum and ileum assessable by endoscopy. The use of
capsule endoscopy and small bowel enteroscopy for diagnosis
of small bowel lymphoma is limited by their inability to obtain
an adequate biopsy for histology. False negativity and inadvertent complications are common. The delay for definitive
operative exploration may result in months of undiagnosed
disease. Unlike malignant carcinomas, systemic chemotherapy
is the standard treatment, and endoscopic ultrasonography
for more precise TMN staging may not be necessary.

Staging, Treatment and Prognosis

The optimal treatment of small bowel lymphoma relies on
both the histology and staging. For each histologic type, the
prognosis is governed by clinical factors. The clinical Ann
Arbor staging (I–IV) is used for nodal Hodgkin's lymphoma.
Attempts have been made to modify it for the staging of

other extra-nodal malignant lymphomas (Table 9.2). Most small bowel lymphomas (80%) are confined to the intestinal area, although liver, pancreatic and peritoneal spread is not uncommon. The clinical prognosis is determined by the International Prognostic Index, which includes the clinical stage, age, LDH level, performance score, and number of extra-nodal sites (score: 0, best prognosis; 5, worst prognosis). The index is derived from patients with diffuse large cell lymphoma treated with curative intent, but has also been verified for other clinical groups, histology and sites. The overall 5-year survival of small bowel lymphoma is around 30–50%, but varies according to the pathology (worse for high-grade histology and much worse for T-cell lineage) and clinical prognostic factors (disease extent and treatment tolerance).

The optimal treatment of small bowel lymphoma has never been determined by prospective clinical trials. For both low-and high-grade lesions, prognosis is worse than that of gastric lymphoma. Operative resection is an important part of the initial management. Up to 80% of the patients would have a bowel resection, either electively or, more commonly, urgently for complications such as perforation, bleeding, and obstruction. But operative intervention may not be beneficial for patients with bulky or disseminated disease. Palliative operative intervention or biopsy are required in 15% and 6%

TABLE 9.2. Staging of gastrointestinal lymphoma by Musshoff modifications of Ann Arbor criteria.

Stage	Definition
Ia	One tumor area without perforation
Ib	Multiple tumors, no perforation
IIa	Gastric or mesenteric nodes involved
IIb	Perforation and adhesions
IIc	Frank peritonitis
III	Widespread thoracic/para-aortic/pelvic nodes
IV	Extra-lymphatic non-adjacent tissue involved

of patients, respectively. Nevertheless, in several multivariate analyses, the ability to perform a complete or de-bulking resection was a favorable prognostic factor. Chemotherapy, either alone or as part of multi-modality treatment, is used for over 90% of patients. Multi-agent chemotherapy (6–8 cycles) gives a synergistic effect and avoids overlapping toxicity. The agents used commonly are cyclophosphamide, anthracycline, vincristine, and steroids. Methotrexate, bleomycin, cytosine arabinoside, and cis-platinum are reserved for second-line treatment. All these regimes may cause gastrointestinal complications that require operative intervention, such as ileus (vincristine), mucositis (methotrexate), gastrointestinal bleeding and wound dehiscence (steroids), pancytopenia causing bleeding and infective typhlitis, acalculous cholecystitis, and peritonitis. Insertion of a central venous catheter is often required for delivery of chemotherapy, blood products, antimicrobials, and parenteral nutrition. For B-cell lymphomas expressing CD20, adding rituximab (anti-CD20) to the chemotherapy gives additional benefit. Radiotherapy can cause ileus and enteritis, but may be useful as adjuvant treatment (5–26%) for obstructive or residual diseases. With operative resection and chemotherapy, over 70% of patients achieve a remission. Relapses, usually extraintestinal, may occur. In patients with relapsing or disseminated disease, autologous or allogenic hematopoietic stem cell transplantation may be considered.

Selected Readings

Azab MB, Henry-Amar M, Rougier P et al. (1989) Prognostic factors in primary gastrointestinal non-Hodgkin's lymphoma. A multivariate analysis, report of 106 cases, and review of the literature. Cancer 64:1208–1217

Koch P, del Valle F, Berdel WE et al. (2001) Primary gastrointestinal non-Hodgkin's lymphoma: I. Anatomic and histologic distribution, clinical features, and survival data of 371 patients registered in the German Multicenter Study GIT NHL 01/92. J Clin Oncol 19: 3861–3873

Koh PK, Horsman JM, Radstone CR et al. (2001) Localised extranodal non-Hodgkin's lymphoma of the gastrointestinal tract: Sheffield Lymphoma Group experience (1989–1998). Int J Oncol 18:743–748

Lee J, Kim WS, Kim K et al. (2004) Intestinal lymphoma: exploration of the prognostic factors and the optimal treatment. Leuk Lymphoma 45:339–344

Liang R, Todd D, Chan TK et al. (1995) Prognostic factors for primary gastrointestinal lymphoma. Hematol Oncol 13:153–163

Lecuit M, Abachin E, Martin A et al. (2004) Immunoproliferative small intestinal disease associated with Campylobacter jejuni. N Engl J Med 350:239–248

Nakamura S, Matsumoto T, Takeshita M et al. (2000) A clinicopathologic study of primary small intestine lym-phoma: prognostic significance of mucosa-associated lymphoid tissue-derived lymphoma. Cancer 88:286–294

Nomura K, Tomikashi K Matsumoto Y et al. (2005) Small bowel non-Hodgkin's lymphoma remaining in complete remission by surgical resection and adjuvant rituximab therapy. World J Gastroenterol 11:4443–4444

Stovroff MC, Coran AG, Hutchinson RJ (1991) The role of surgery in American Burkitt's lymphoma in children. J Pediatr Surg 26:1235–1238

10
Carcinoid of the Small Bowel

John R. Porterfield and David R. Farley

Pearls and Pitfalls

- The ileum harbors ~85% of small bowel carcinoid (SBC) neoplasms.
- Vague GI complaints are present typically for years prior to diagnosis.
- Less than 10% of SBCs present with "carcinoid syndrome."
- Laparotomy detects the majority of SBCs; a pre-op diagnosis is uncommon.
- Approximately 90% of patients with SBCs have evidence of metastases at exploration.
- Approximately 30% have multicentric disease.
- Most SBCs are <2 cm in diameter.
- Oncologic resection with primary anastomosis represents optimal therapy.
- Overall recurrence rate is 80%.

Background

It has been nearly 140 years since carcinoid neoplasms of the small bowel were first described. In 1867, Theodore Langhans described these lesions as *Drusenpolyp im Ileum* and Lubrarsch described "little carcinomata" in two patients in

K.I. Bland et al. (eds.), *Surgery of the Small Bowel*,
DOI: 10.1007/978-1-84996-372-5_10,
© Springer-Verlag London Limited 2011

1888. In 1907, the term Karzinoid was coined by Oberndorfer due to the morphologic similarities with adenocarcinomas; he was mistaken in his belief that these neoplasms were benign which we now know is not the case. Carcinoid neoplasms have been described throughout the entire gastrointestinal tract and foregut structures, which includes the thymus, bronchi, and lung. These neoplasms were classified in 1963 by Williams and Sandler according to their embryologic development and blood supply as foregut (celiac axis), midgut (superior mesenteric artery), and hindgut (inferior mesenteric artery) regions.

Carcinoid neoplasms arise from the neuroendocrine Kulchitsky cells found in the base of the crypts of Lieberkuhn and are a part of the APUD (amine precursor uptake and decarboxylation) system (Fig. 10.1). These totipotent cells are capable of secreting multiple metabolically active hormones and biogenic amines, such as serotonin, histamine, tachykinins, dopamine, substance P, prostaglandins, and others. Serotonin, the most commonly secreted substance from small bowel carcinoids, is derived from its precursor 5-hydroxytryptophan and is metabolized to 5-hydroxyindole acetic acid (5-HIAA) excreted and quantifiable in urine.

Small bowel carcinoids are the second most common small intestinal neoplasm (#1 ¼ adenocarcinomas). Thus, it is important to have a thorough understanding of the surgical and medical management of these unique neoplasms, because they are often discovered incidentally.

Clinical Presentation

Small bowel carcinoids (SBCs) present typically in the sixth or seventh decades of life with a slight male predominance. These neoplasms are nearly twice as common in black vs. white patients (incidence of 9.2 vs. 5.4 per million, respectively) according to a recent evaluation of the SEER (Surveillance, Epidemiology, and End Results) program. The most common anatomic part of small bowel is the ileum which harbors 85%. The typical presentation is 2–20 years of nonspecific

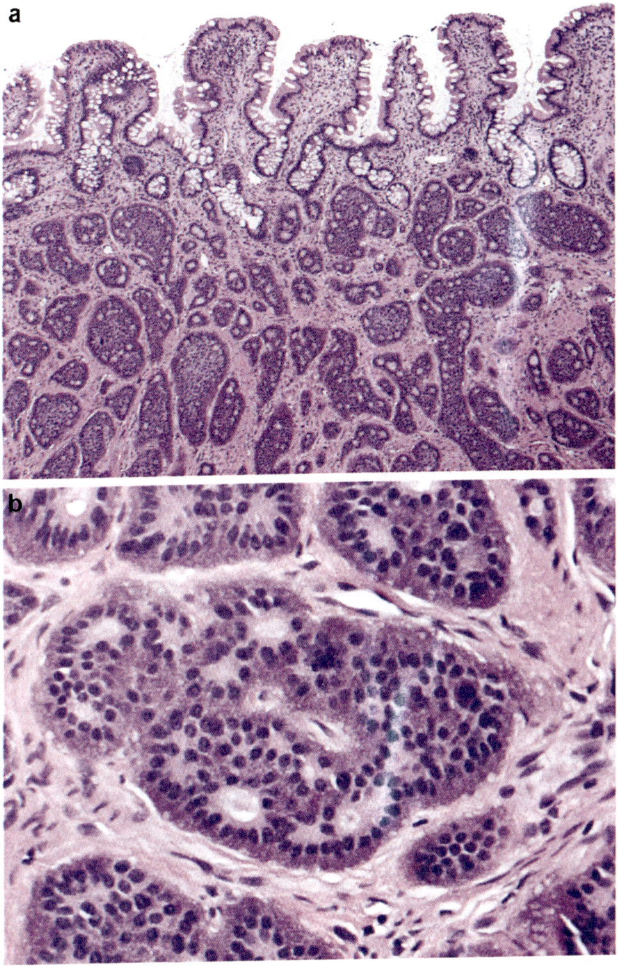

FIGURE 10.1. Low and high power H+E views of submucosal small bowel carcinoid neoplasm.

gastrointestinal symptoms, abdominal pain, or intestinal obstruction. Patients have often been labeled with a variety of diagnoses, including irritable bowel syndrome, Crohn's disease, adhesive obstruction, lymphoma, and colitis. Less than

10% of patients present with true carcinoid syndrome characterized by cutaneous flushing, usually of the face, that cycles as quickly as every 10–30 min and begins resolution centrally. These episodes are associated often with tachycardia, diarrhea, sweating, and hypotension. SBCs may present with intestinal ischemia, an abdominal mass, or hepatomegaly, but this presentation is extremely rare. Because these submucosal neoplasms grow slowly, they do not cause symptoms typically until the disease has spread beyond the wall of the intestine, and, thus, greater than 90% are metastatic at initial presentation (Fig. 10.2). Because SBCs are also multicentric in 30% of patients, a meticulous exploration of the entire small bowel is necessary once the diagnosis is suspected.

These unique neoplasms can secrete a broad range of metabolically active substances that maybe triggered by serotonin-rich foods such as coffee, cheese, alcohol, or exercise. Even patients with significant tumor burden may have minimal

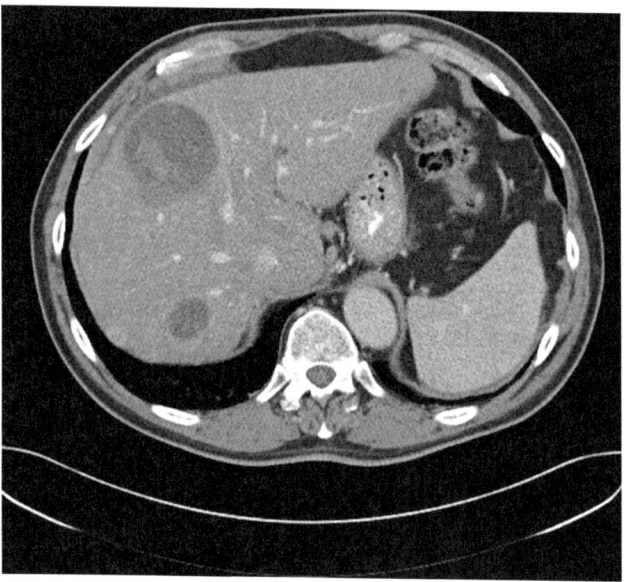

FIGURE 10.2. Computed tomography with extensive hepatic metastases from a primary small bowel carcinoid neoplasm.

symptoms and evade detection through serologic testing because of their rapid "first pass" metabolism of these vasoactive substances in the liver. It is not until the secretory burden overwhelms the metabolic capabilities of the liver or the hormones are secreted directly into the systemic circulation via the hepatic veins from hepatic implants that the symptoms manifest. When carcinoid syndrome is present, the astute physician should also suspect the presence of nonendocrine malignancies found in 29% of patients with SBCs. Colorectal adenomas and carcinomas are associated most frequently with SBCs, but cancers of the breast, stomach, and lung are also seen. Therefore, chest radiography, mammography, and upper and lower gastrointestinal endoscopy are useful preoperatively.

Diagnosis

While numerous preoperative studies aid in the diagnosis of SBCs, the vast majority of patients are diagnosed in the operating room. In order for the diagnosis to be made preoperatively there must be a high index of suspicion with application of multiple, semi-confirmatory tests. An increased 24 hurine 5-HIAA is the most reliable preoperative finding, yet nearly half of patients have normal levels preoperatively. Similarly, plasma serotonin, substance P, neurotensin, neurokin A, and neuropeptide K are all measurable with immunofluorescent neuropeptide assays, but their sensitivity is low because most such substances are not increased in the majority of patients. Unfortunately, the one marker that seems to be increased consistently, chromogranin A, is not specific to carcinoid neoplasms.

Because most carcinoid neoplasms are small (<2cm), visualization with preoperative imaging is difficult. Contrast studies of the small bowel are usually unrewarding but may demonstrate one or more of the following findings: (1) solitary or multiple submucosal lesions; (2) mesenteric infiltration or retraction with or without lymphadenopathy; or (3) polypoid, mucosal-based masses. When these findings are present, the differential diagnosis includes SBCs, small bowel adenocarcinoma, lymphoma, Kaposi's sarcoma, and metastatic melanoma.

Even with the advent of high resolution computed tomography (CT) and magnetic resonance imaging (MRI), the primary neoplasms of SBCs are often undetectable; these cross-sectional imaging modalities with selective angiography, however, are beneficial in depicting the extent of metastatic disease and potential resectability. Lymph node metastases are often bulky and cause a swirling desmoplastic reaction in the base of the mesentery which accounts for the symptoms of ischemia due to the intense fibrosis and mass effect on the mesenteric vasculature (Fig. 10.3). Hepatic metastases are hypervascular, yet both contrast-enhanced CT and MRI tend to underestimate the burden of disease appreciable intraoperatively and pathologically (Fig. 10.4).

Somatostatin receptor scintigraphy (OctreoScan) has been shown repeatedly to be the most sensitive imaging modality (~85%) for detecting carcinoid neoplasms. This noninvasive imaging modality relies on the density of somatostatin receptors and is able to detect tumors of ~1 cm diameter. The

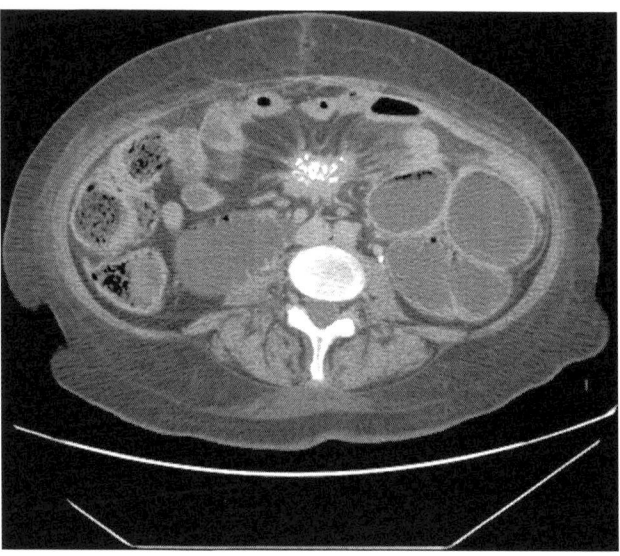

FIGURE 10.3. Computed tomography of the abdomen with dense mesenteric fibrosis.

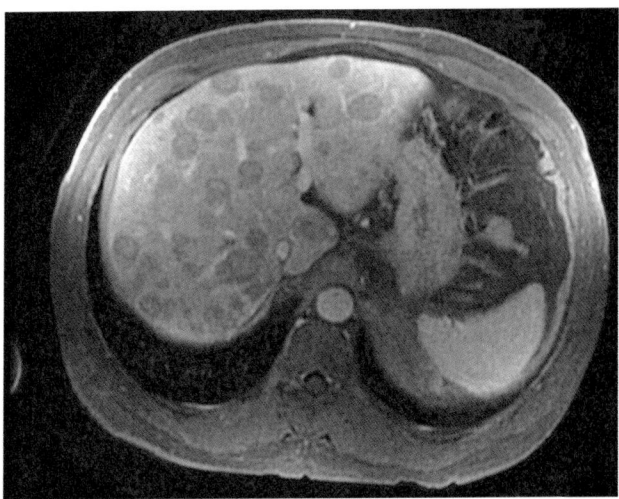

FIGURE 10.4. Magnetic resonance imaging of the liver with extensive hepatic metastases from a primary small bowel carcinoid neoplasm.

OctreoScan is not, however, able to determine the size of the neoplasms, because the image produced is a reflection of the density of the somatostatin receptors which may or may not correlate with the actual tumor size. Similarly, scintigraphy cannot detect those neoplasms that do not express the somatostatin receptors. Additionally, the first pass affect of the somatostatin analogue causes physiologic enhancement of the genitourinary system and spleen, which may produce sufficient background signal to hide lesions in the left upper quadrant and mid abdomen. Its use intraoperatively to guide or quantify the adequacy of resection is still under evaluation.

Preoperative Management

When the diagnosis is obtained preoperatively, it is crucial to recognize the characteristic symptoms of carcinoid syndrome to minimize morbidity and potential mortality. Asymptomatic patients may proceed to a curative resection with minimal preparation. In contrast, symptomatic patients are at risk for carcinoid crisis which is hallmarked by profound hypotension or bronchospasm during induction of general anesthesia or intraoperative manipulation of the neoplasm. The goal for preoperative management is to render the patients symptom-free with use of a somatostatin analogue. The majority (~75%) of symptomatic patients are able to be suppressed with oct-reotide at dosages ranging from 50 to 500 mg subcutaneously three times each day. The dosage should be titrated in accordance with symptom control. Longer acting somatostatin analogues are available (lanreotide and Sandostatin LAR) which allow dosing every 2 or 4 weeks, respectively. At the time of operation, previously suppressed patients should also receive a subcutaneous bolus of octreotide with induction of anesthesia and an additional 100 mg of octreotide should be immediately available to be administered intravenously in the setting of a carcinoid crisis. Additionally, the anesthesia team needs to be prepared to treat octreotide-induced brady-cardia and heart block in the setting of a carcinoid resection.

The second facet regarding the preoperative evaluation is to exclude carcinoid heart disease. This rare but important complication occurs in approximately 5% of patients with SBCs and is characterized by heart murmurs and/or right-sided heart failure. Patients with hepatic metastases are at the highest risk for tricuspid insufficiency, because the secretions from the hepatic metastases are fed unaltered directly into the hepatic veins and thus directly to the heart. Transesophageal echocardiography should complete the preoperative evaluation, and carcinoid heart disease should be treated prior to abdominal exploration.

Operative Management

SBCs tend to be more aggressive and have a greater ultimate risk of death than carcinoids found in other locations. Given that these neoplasms are multicentric (30%) and usually (90%) metastatic, resection should proceed only after meticulous abdominal inspection with the goal of rendering the patient disease-free (Fig. 10.5). The primary tumor should be resected

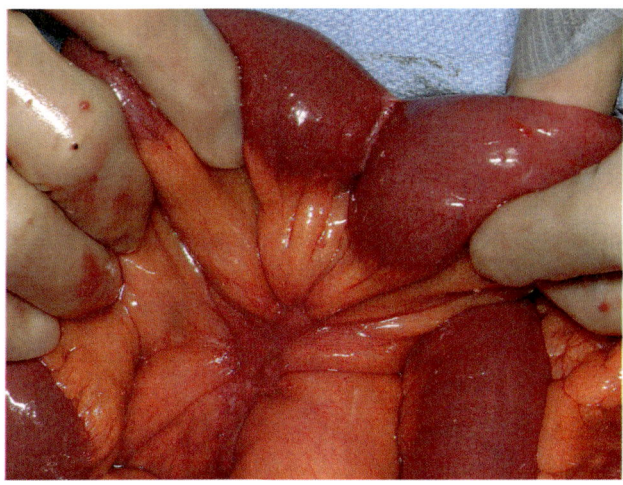

FIGURE 10.5. Gross photograph of ileal carcinoid. Note the small primary neoplasm and the sclerosing mesenteric response.

with a wide tumor-free margin and excised en bloc with the maximal mesenteric resection to maintain an adequate vascular supply to the remaining bowel. Debulking of lymphadenopathy may be beneficial in delaying the mesenteric desmoplastic reaction and subsequent bowel obstruction or ischemia.

In the setting of hepatic metastases, palliative cytoreductive resection is beneficial for symptom control and is associated with increased survival when 90% of the tumor burden is removed. Sequential hepatic artery embolization may be considered when resection or in situ destruction (ablation techniques) is not a viable option to improve symptoms and slow the progression of the disease.

Postoperative Care

Care after a small bowel resection for a carcinoid neoplasm should be routine. The nasogastric tube is discontinued the evening of operation or the following morning. A liquid diet is initiated and advanced rapidly to a soft diet as tolerated. In patients who are asymptomatic preoperatively, there is no indication for postoperative somatostatin or other ongoing therapy. In contrast, patients who were symptomatic postoperatively should be continued on suppressive therapy. If there was significant debulking of the neoplasm, the dosage of somatostatin should be reduced to the lowest therapeutic dose.

In our practice, the timing of follow-up is driven by the clinical suspicion for recurrence at the time of resection. When the primary neoplasm and its associated nodal basin are resected without evidence of distant disease, patients are re-evaluated in 4–6 months. In the setting of distant disease where greater than 90% of the tumor burden was resected, we prefer a baseline set of imaging and laboratory studies within 2 months. Serial 24 h urine 5-HIAA concentrations and Chromogranin A levels are followed at each visit. We use CT for evaluation of the remaining small bowel and its associated mesentery. The best imaging for hepatic metastasis is MRI, while OctreoScans are used to survey for disease that may have spread beyond the abdomen.

In the setting of metastatic disease, many treatment options are available, but there is no magic bullet. Single agent chemotherapeutics (5-fluorouracil, doxorubicin, actinomycin D, dacarbazine, and streptozocin) have been little benefit. Combination chemotherapy, using streptozocin and 5-FU (cyclophosphamide), produces biochemical and tumor response rates in only 8–25% of patients. No single or combination chemotherapy has demonstrated a response rate of greater than 15% when using the criteria of 50% reduction in bidimensionally measurable disease. This slow-growing neoplasm is essentially chemoresistant.

Carcinoid neoplasms are also usually radioresistant, but external beam therapy has been beneficial in symptom control in the brain, bone, and near the spinal cord, where local growth causes clinically significant pain or neurologic deficits. Recent advances in systemic receptor-targeted and metabolically directed radiotherapy have been utilized for unresectable patients. These agents consists of 131I-MIBG or radiolabeled somatostatin analogues. Overall response rates range from 10% to 20%. The most likely use of these agents will be to slow the rate of progression to maintain a stable tumor burden.

While carcinoids from other regions have long-term survival, the overall 5-year survival for patients with SBC is 60%. When the disease presents with only regional disease, the 5-year survival is 90%; when inoperable liver metastases are present, the 5-year survival is approximately 50% and decreases further to 42% when there is accompanying mesenteric adenopathy. Therefore, when radical hepatic resection and metastasectomy is feasible technically, an aggressive resection should be pursued because the 5-year survival may extend to 70%.

Summary

Carcinoid neoplasms are the second most common small bowel neoplasm and are often discovered incidentally due to their myriad of clinical presentations. To establish the diagnosis preoperatively, physicians must be sensitized to the possibility of their presence when caring for patients with chronic, vague, and insidious abdominal symptoms. There are many investigative studies that may aid in the diagnosis, but none is pathognomonic or highly sensitive. An aggressive operative approach should be pursued; SBCs should be resected with wide margins to include the maximal mesenteric nodal basin. Patients with metastatic disease may be candidates for resection or image-guided destruction of the neoplasms, in light of the limited chemotherapeutic and radiotherapy options. Follow-up should be focused on detection of recurrent symptoms and imaging to detect treatable metastatic disease.

Selected Readings

Dilger JA, Rho EH, Que FG et al. (2004) Octreotide-induced bradycardia and heart block during surgical resection of a carcinoid tumor. Anesth Analg 98:318–320

Hellman P, Lundstrom T, Ohrvall U et al. (2002) Effect of surgery on the outcome of midgut carcinoid disease with lymph node and liver metastases. World J Surg 26:991–997

Kerstrom G, Hellman P, Hessman O (2005) Midgut carcinoid tumours: surgical treatment and prognosis. Baillieres Best PractRes Clin Gastroenterol 19:717–728

Modlin IM, Kidd M, Latich I et al. (2005) Current status of gastrointestinal carcinoids. Gastroenterology 128:1717–1751

Modlin IM, Lye KD, Kidd M (2003) A 5-decade analysis of 13,715 carcinoid tumors. Cancer 97:934–959

Oberndorfer S (1907) Karzenoide Tumoren des Dünn-darms. Frankfurt Zeitschr Pathol 1:426–432

Que FG, Nagorney DM, Batts KP et al. (1995) Hepatic resection for metastatic neuroendocrine carcinomas. Am J Surg 169:36–42

Williams ED, SandlerM (1963) The classification of carcinoid tumours. Lancet 1:238–239

Zar N, Garmo H, Holmberg L et al. (2004) Long-term survival of patients with small intestinal carcinoid tumors. World J Surg 28:1163–1168

11

Stromal Tumors of the Small Bowel

Sherry J. Lim and Peter W.T. Pisters

Pearls and Pitfalls

- High index of suspicion of small bowel malignancy is necessary for early detection.
- Favorable prognostic factors: no tumor rupture, localized lesion, low-grade neoplasm, and tumor <5 cm.
- CT can often aid in differentiation between sarcoma, adenocarcinoma, carcinoid, and lymphoma.
- Primary therapy for patients with localized sarcomas and gastrointestinal stromal tumors (GISTs) is operative resection when feasible. At present, there is no defined role for adjuvant or neoadjuvant imatinib mesylate.
- Lymphadenectomy is not required for operative treatment of sarcomas.
- Care must be taken to avoid tumor rupture during resection.
- GISTs are almost always positive for CD117 (KIT), frequently for CD34, occasionally for SMA, and rarely for S-100 or desmin.
- Standard, first-line therapy for metastatic or unresectable GIST is imatinib mesylate.
- Second line therapy for imatinib resistant or intolerant GIST is sunitinib.

K.I. Bland et al. (eds.), *Surgery of the Small Bowel*,
DOI: 10.1007/978-1-84996-372-5_11,
© Springer-Verlag London Limited 2011

Introduction

Although the small intestine constitutes more than 75% of the intestinal tract, small bowel malignancies are rare. Indeed, small bowel neoplasms account for only 2–3% of digestive system cancers and less than 1% of all cancers diagnosed annually. According to the American Cancer Society, 6,000 cases of small bowel cancers are expected to be diagnosed in 2006. This number, however, may be a significant under-estimation of the true incidence of small bowel malignancies. The true incidence of gastrointestinal stromal tumors (GISTs) is unknown in the United States, but based on population studies completed in Europe, the true incidence of GISTs may be as high as 5,000–6,000 annually, of which 30% occur in the small bowel.

Adenocarcinomas are the most common small bowel malignancies (5.9 cases per million persons; 45% of all small bowel malignancies), followed by carcinoids (5.5 cases per million; 30% of all small bowel malignancies), lymphomas (3 cases per million; 15% of all small bowel malignancies), and sarcomas (1.7 cases per million; 10% of all small bowel malig-nancies). Unlike adenocarcinomas of the small intestine but similar to small bowel carcinoids and lymphomas, small bowel sarcomas are found most commonly in the jejunum and ileum; only 10% of small bowel sarcomas occur in the duodenum. This chapter will focus on the incidence, diagnosis, as well as current treatment recommendations for small bowel sarco-mas. Particular attention to management of GISTs will be emphasized, because a treatment algorithm for this disease entity continue to evolve with new treatment paradigms.

Classification

Sarcomas develop from cells derived from the mesoderm. Mesenchymal cells can differentiate into fibroblasts, myo-blasts, lipoblasts, chondroblasts, osteoblasts, etc., which then differentiate into the various mature cell lines. Unlike epidermal malignancies, where the extent of tumor invasion and the presence of metastasis predict the course of the disease and its treatment, the behavior of sarcomas can be predicted by the tumor grade based on morphologic criteria and classification based on cell of origin. Therefore, the histologic classification is important in defining the natural history, estimating prognosis, and selecting therapy.

   Small bowel sarcomas, like other sarcomas, are classified on the basis of histology, cell of origin, and dominant cell pattern. Small bowel sarcomas include smooth muscle tumors (leiomyomas, leiomyosarcomas, leiomyoblastoma), neoplasms of the peripheral nerve sheath (schwannoma, paraganglioma), fibrous neoplasms (desmoid tumor, fibrosarcoma), and mixed neoplasms (Table 11.1). Excluding GISTs (described below), the most common sarcomas of the small intestine are leiomyosarcomas (75%), followed by epithelioid leiomyosarcomas (7%), Kaposi's sarcomas (4%), sarcomas not otherwise specified (4%), and spindle cell sarcomas (3%). The diverse cellular morphology as well as the overlapping histology of sarcomas, makes classification based on

TABLE 11.1. Subtypes of gastrointestinal sarcomas.

Leiomyoma

Leiomyosarcoma

Leiomyoblastoma

Schwann cell neoplasm

Paraganglioma

Desmoid tumor

Mesenchymal tumor

Mixed cell sarcoma

Stromal tumor of uncertain malignant potential

Gastrointestinal autonomic nerve tumor (GANT)

Gastrointestinal stromal tumor (GIST)

Fibrosarcoma

morphology alone difficult. Therefore, immunohistochemistry has become an important adjunct to diagnosis (and eventual treatment).

Historically, GISTs were thought to be derived from smooth muscle cells, nerve cells, or other mesenchyme-derived cells; and as such, these neoplasms were classified previously as leiomyoblastomas, leiomyomas, or leiomyosarcomas. Since the 1990s, GISTs have been considered a distinct pathologic entity. These mesenchymal tumors result from neoplastic transformation of the interstitial cells of Cajal, which function as intestinal pacemaker cells. Mutation occurs in the c-kit protooncogene, which encodes for the type III receptor tyrosine kinase KIT. The most frequent mutation causing GISTs occurs in exon 11, which encodes the intracellular juxtamembranous region of the receptor. Other exon mutations have been observed, particularly in exon 9, with small bowel GISTs. These mutated KIT receptors are activated constitutively, leading to neoplastic development and progression. Advances in the understanding of GIST biology were instrumental in the development of imatinib as a targeted therapeutic tool.

Presentation

The mean age of patients with small bowel sarcomas is 53 years, while the mean age of patients with GISTs is 63 years; 80% of all GISTs are diagnosed after age 50. For all small bowel sarcomas, including GISTs, there is a slight male predominance (~55%). The majority of small bowel sarcomas are reported in white, non-Hispanic patients (85%). Among the ethnic groups, African-Americans have a higher prevalence in both small bowel sarcomas and GISTs.

The symptoms of GISTs and other small bowel sarcomas at presentation depend on the size and location of the tumor and include vague abdominal pain, bleeding, increased abdominal girth, or, rarely, obstruction. Because most of the clinical symptoms that occur are nonspecific in nature, diagnosis is often delayed. Furthermore, many patients with small bowel sarcomas are asymptomatic, and the neoplasms are diagnosed incidentally as a result of imaging studies performed for another condition or at the time of unrelated laparotomy.

Diagnosis

The differential diagnosis of a small bowel mass includes adenocarcinoma, carcinoid, lymphoma, malignant melanoma, GIST, or sarcomas such as leiomyoma, leiomyosarcoma, malignant peripheral nerve sheath tumor, and schwannoma, as well as benign conditions such as fibromatosis and inflammatory myofibroblastic tumor. Once a small bowel mass is found or suspected, contrast-enhanced computed tomography (CT) is recommended and may facilitate differentiation between adenocarcinoma, carcinoid, and lymphoma. Importantly, radiographic findings of malignancy, such as invasion to adjacent structures or distant metastasis, may be identified. On CT, most small bowel sarcomas, including GISTs, appear as well-defined extraluminal or intramural masses with varying attenuation depending on the size. Small tumors are typically enhancing homogeneous masses, while larger tumors (>6 cm) may have central areas of necrosis or hemorrhage. In the small intestine, sarcomas often appear as intraluminal masses or intraluminal polyps and may show extension into the adjacent mesentery. Sarcomas can often be distinguished from adenocarcinomas and lymphomas, because adenocarcinomas are usually annular lesions, while lymphomas are accompanied typically by lymphadenopathy. Radiographically, additional tests, such as upper gastrointestinal series with small bowel follow-through and enteroclysis, may be necessary to distinguish carcinoid from other small bowel malignancies.

If a pretreatment diagnosis is required, a biopsy can often be performed endoscopically or percutaneously. In addition to histopathologic evaluation, immunohistochemical characterization of the tumor can assist with classification of small bowel sarcomas. This is particularly true for diagnosis of GISTs. Immunohistochemical evaluation has become essential in the

TABLE 11.2. Immunophenotypes of GIST and other spindle cell neoplasms of the GI tract (Adapted from Fletcher et al., 2002).

Tumor	KIT (CD117)	CD34	Smooth muscle actin	S-100 protein	Desmin
GIST	+++	++	+	+	Very rare
Leiomyosarcoma	–	+	+	Rare	+
Schwannoma	–	+	–	+	–
Fibromatosis	–	Rare	+	–	Rare

GIST, gastrointestinal stromal tumor; GI, gastrointestinal.

diagnosis of GISTs and should include staining for CD117 (KIT), CD34, smooth muscle actin (SMA), desmin, and S-100 to distinguish between GISTs, smooth muscle neoplasms (leiomyoma and leiomyosarcoma), schwannoma, and fibromatosis (Table 11.2). In addition to CD117 positivity (95%), GISTs may demonstrate immunopositivity for CD34 (65%), SMA (35%), and S-100 (5%). True KIT-positive GISTs, however, are rarely positive for desmin.

Histologically, there are three categories of GISTs: spindle cell type (70%), epithelioid type (20%), and mixed type. These neoplasms are classified as very low-, low-, intermediate-, or high-risk based on anatomic site (gastric versus small bowel), size, and mitotic rate. A commonly used classification system is outlined in Table 11.3.

TABLE 11.3. Potential malignant behavior of small bowel GISTs (Adapted from Miettinen et al., 2002).

	Size (cm)	Mitoses per 50 HPF
Benign	≤2	≤5
Intermediate	>2–5	≤5
Malignant	>5	>5

HPF, high-power fields; GIST, gastrointestinal stromal tumor.

Prognosis

The 5-year, disease-specific survival rate in patients with small bowel sarcomas is about 35%, with a median, disease-specific survival duration of 32 months. Factors associated with a better prognosis are complete (R0) operative resection without tumor rupture, localized lesion, low tumor grade, and size <5 cm. Despite aggressive surgical resection, patients with tumor rupture, contiguous organ invasion, and high tumor grade are at increased risk for recurrence.

Treatment for Non-GISTs Sarcomas

Complete operative resection is the mainstay of therapy for localized disease. Extensive lymphadenectomy is not indicated, because lymph node metastases are seen only rarely in sarcomas; however, en-bloc resection of the lesions to achieve tumor-free margins should be attempted for potentially curative resections. Localized disease and complete surgical resection are independent variables in overall survival (50 months vs. 15 months). Even when contiguous organ involvement or peritoneal implants were encountered at the time of operation, the ability to achieve complete resection conferred an overall survival advantage (36 months vs. 21 months). For high-grade sarcomas, unresectable lesions, and recurrent disease, a protocol-based treatment should be offered to patients in attempt to downstage the disease or convert an unresectable neoplasm to a resectable one.

Treatment for GISTs

Though the treatment algorithm continues to evolve, current treatment of primary and metastatic GISTs involves a combination of operative resection, imatinib mesylate, and close monitoring (Fig. 11.1).

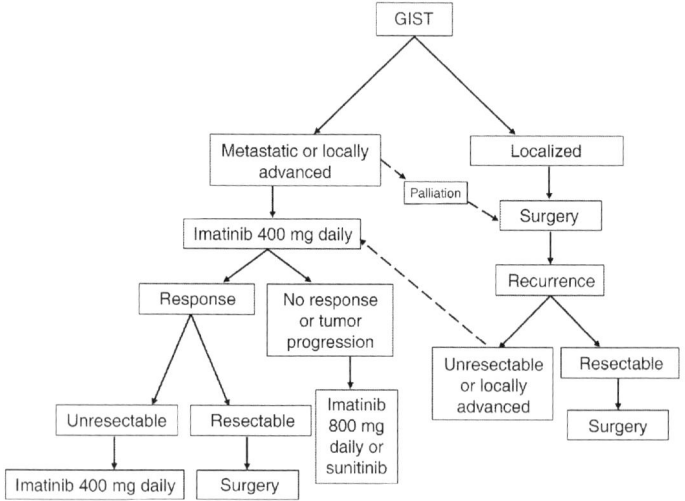

FIGURE 11.1. Treatment algorithm for GIST.

Operative Therapy

Like other sarcomas, complete resection is the primary treatment for patients with localized GISTs. GISTs can be friable and fragile, so care must be taken to avoid rupture or tumor shedding during resection, because this has been linked to an increased risk of peritoneal recurrence. Although some GISTs appear large on CT, they may have a small stalk or base, because these neoplasms tend to grow in an extraluminal fashion without invasion of adjacent structures (Fig. 11.2).

The goal of operative resection is to achieve macroscopically and microscopically negative surgical margins (R0). Therefore, if the neoplasm is locally advanced at the time of surgery, en bloc resection of adjacent involved organs may be required. In contrast to adenocarcinomas, lymph node metastases are rare in GISTs, and thus, lymphadenectomy is not warranted.

In a study by Dematteo et al., 200 patients with GISTs were evaluated for operative resection. A complete R0 resection was achieved in 80 of the 93 patients with localized primary GISTs and in 34 of the 94 patients with metastatic or locally recurrent disease. Patients with localized GISTs who

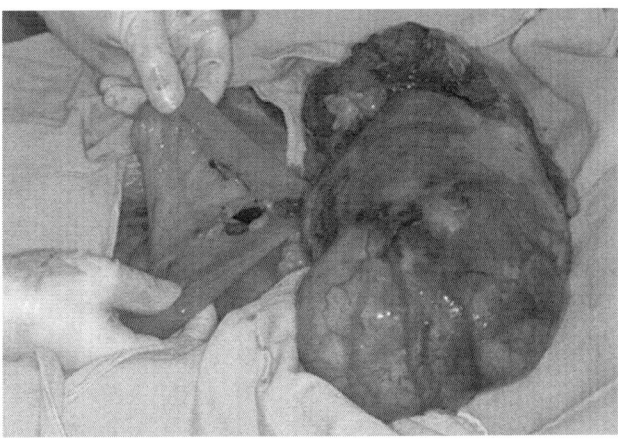

FIGURE 11.2. Large mid-jejunal GIST with a small base and no evidence of local invasion to adjacent organs at the time of exploration.

underwent complete R0 resection had a 5-year, disease-specific survival of 54%, with a median survival of 66 months. In contrast, patients with incomplete resection or unresectable neoplasms had a median survival of only 22 months. A subset of patients with metastatic disease who underwent complete resection had a median survival of 16 months versus only 5 months for patients who had an incomplete resection or unresectable disease.

Disease recurrence is usually intraabdominal and is seen first in the liver or on the peritoneal surface. Extraabdominal metastases may occur later in the course of the disease. The treatment of recurrent disease usually involves primary therapy with imatinib mesylate in conjunction with selective use of operative resection.

Imatinib

Primary Therapy for Metastases

Imatinib mesylate (Gleevec), which was used first in patients with chronic myeloid leukemia, is a small molecule

inhibitor of ABL-kinase, KIT, and platelet-derived growth
factor A and B. Imatinib binds to the intracellular portion of
KIT and inhibits cell signaling. When imatinib is used to
treat metastatic GISTs, partial responses are achieved in
50% of patients, and stable disease is achieved in an additional 30%. The 2-year, overall-survival rate is reported to
be 75% in patients with metastatic GISTs treated with imatinib. The current standard dose of imatinib is 400 mg daily.
Patients whose neoplasm progresses while receiving the
standard dose are considered for a dose escalation or are
offered second-line therapy with sunitinib (Sutent). Even
though imatinib is well tolerated by patients, most patients
experience some adverse effects, including edema (74%),
nausea (52%), diarrhea (45%), myalgia (40%), and abdominal pain (26%).

Adjuvant Therapy

Currently, there is no defined role for adjuvant imatinib
therapy after complete resection of localized GIST. Phase II
and III clinical trials are under way to better define the possible role of adjuvant imatinib. The American College of
Surgeons Oncology Group (ACOSOG) is conducting a sin-
gle-arm, phase II clinical trial (Z9000) of adjuvant imatinib
for patients with completely resected high-risk GISTs. Accrual
began in June 2001 and was completed in September 2003
with enrollment of 110 patients. Primary and secondary end
points being evaluated are overall survival and recurrence,
respectively. A report of the primary end-point analysis is
expected in late 2006.

Also under way is ACOSOG Z9001, a phase III, randomized, double-blind trial of adjuvant imatinib versus placebo
after resection of localized GISTs. Inclusion criteria for this
study include tumor size 3 cm, CD117-positivity, and complete (R0) operative resection. Patients are assigned ran-
domly to receive either imatinib (400 mg daily) or placebo
for 1 year. The primary end point is disease-free survival

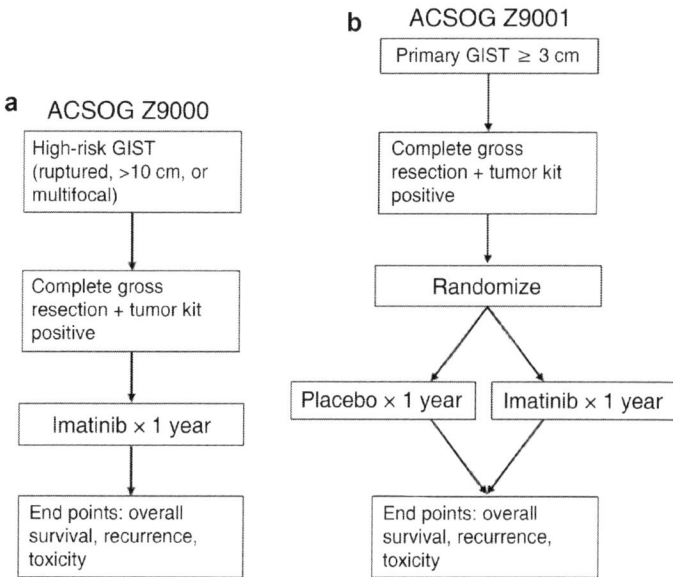

FIGURE 11.3. Clinical trials of adjuvant therapy for GIST conducted by the American College of Surgeons Oncology Group (ACOSOG). (**a**) Z9000 is a phase II trial for patients with completely resected high-risk GISTs. (**b**) Z9001 is a phase III randomized, double-blind study of adjuvant imatinib versus placebo for patients with completely resected primary GISTs 3cm.

(Fig. 11.3). In addition, a European, phase III trial (EORTC 62024) is evaluating 2 years of adjuvant imatinib (400 mg daily) compared with observation (Fig. 11.4).

The results of these trials will provide important information on the toxicities of imatinib in a setting of the adjuvant therapy and will define whether there is any clinical benefit to 1 or 2 years of adjuvant imatinib. In the absence of prospective, randomized trials supporting use of imatinib after complete operative resection, there is no present role for adjuvant imatinib treatment outside of clinical trials.

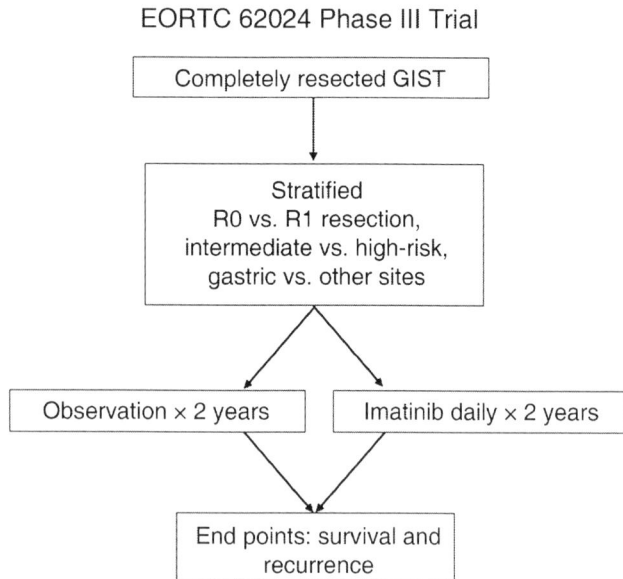

FIGURE 11.4. A phase III randomized study of adjuvant imatinib versus placebo following complete surgical resection of GIST by the European Organization for Research and Treatment of Cancer (EORTC 62024).

Neoadjuvant Therapy

There is also currently no defined role for preoperative (neo-adjuvant) therapy with imatinib. Preoperative imatinib, how-ever, may warrant consideration in specific patient subgroups, including patients with large rectal GISTs and patients with large, locally advanced primary neoplasms. In these unique situations, imatinib-related responses may improve the R0 resection rate or facilitate organ preservation.

At the moment, there are no randomized trials evaluating preoperative imatinib treatment. The Radiation Therapy Oncology Group has an ongoing, phase II trial (S0132) evalu-ating pre-and postoperative imatinib for patients with local-ized or recurrent GISTs. The protocol involves 8 weeks of preoperative imatinib followed by resection and postoperative imatinib for 2 years. The end points are tumor response to imatinib therapy and disease-free survival. This trial will provide insight into the feasibility and toxicities of preoperative therapy with imatinib.

Selected Readings

DeMatteo RP, Lewis JJ, Leung D et al. (2000) Two hundred gastrointestinal stromal tumors: recurrence patterns and prognostic factors for survival. Ann Surg 231:51–58

Fletcher CD, Berman JJ, Corless C et al. (2002) Diagnosis of gastrointestinal stromal tumors: a consensus approach. Hum Pathol 33:459–465

Gold JS, DeMatteo RP (2006) Combined surgical and molecular therapy: the gastrointestinal stromal tumor model. Ann Surg 244:176–184

Hirota S, Isozaki K, Moriyama Y et al. (1998) Gain-of-function mutations of c-kit in human gastrointestinal stromal tumors. Science 279:577–580

Howe JR, Karnell LH, Scott-Conner C (2001) Small bowel sarcoma: analysis of survival from the National Cancer Data Base. Ann Surg Oncol 8:496–508

Kosmadakis N, Visvardis EE, Kartsaklis P et al. (2005) The role of surgery in the management of gastrointestinal stromal tumors (GISTs) in the era of imatinib mesylate effectiveness. Surg Oncol 14:75–84

Miettinen M, El-Rifai WE, Sorbin LH et al. (2002) Evaluation of malignancy and prognosis of gastrointestinal stromal tumors: a review. Hum Pathol 33:478–483

Ng EH, Pollock RE, Munsell MF et al. (1992) Prognostic factors influencing survival in gastrointestinal leiomyo-sarcomas. Implications for surgical management and staging. Ann Surg 215:68–77

Van Glabbeke M, Verweij J, Casali PG et al. (2005) Initial and late resistance to imatinib in advanced gastrointestinal stromal tumors are predicted by different prognostic factors: a European Organization for Research and Treatment of Cancer-Italian Sarcoma Group-Australasian Gastrointestinal Trials Group study. J Clin Oncol 23:5795–5804

Part III
Gastrointestinal Bleeding

12
Upper Gastrointestinal Hemorrhage: Diagnosis and Treatment

Joaquim Gama-Rodrigues, Igor Proscurshim, and Carlos Eduardo Jacob

Pearls and Pitfalls

- Patients with acute upper GI bleeding require aggressive resuscitation.
- Patients with recent or active bleeding need a large bore, intravenous line during the initial evaluation.
- ALWAYS attempt endoscopic control for upper GI bleeding.
- In elderly patients, the hematocrit should be kept above 30%, while in young healthy patients, above 20%.
- Patients that require monitoring should be admitted to an intensive care unit.
- Peptic ulcer is the most common cause of upper GI bleeding.
- Signs of chronic liver disease should be sought.
- All patients with suspected or proven upper GI bleeding require a panendoscopy with the purpose of diagnosis and potentially therapy.
- For occult GI bleeding, diagnosis of the site and cause may require repeated endoscopic examinations, enteroscopy,

K.I. Bland et al. (eds.), *Surgery of the Small Bowel*,
DOI: 10.1007/978-1-84996-372-5_12,
© Springer-Verlag London Limited 2011

video capsule endoscopy, barium contrast series, enteroclysis, angiography, and RBC-tagged radionucleotide scan.

- Aggressive therapy with proton pump inhibitors combined
  with antibiotics to eradicate *Helicobacter pylori* infection
  may be effective in controlling peptic ulcer bleeding.
- Hemodynamically unstable patients or those with ongoing
  bleeding should be considered for immediate operative
  intervention.
- Gastric resection or vagotomy has a relatively high rate of
  morbidity and rebleeding.
- Try to avoid operative intervention in patients who are
  candidates for liver transplantation.

Upper Gastrointestinal Hemorrhage – Diagnosis and Treatment

Upper gastrointestinal (GI) bleeding is a common condition
that obligates a high morbidity and health care burden. The
most common causes of upper gastrointestinal bleeding are
peptic ulcer, gastroesophageal varices, arteriovenous malformations, Mallory-Weiss tears, erosive gastritis, and neoplasms,
both benign and malignant. Patients with upper GI bleeding
may present with hematemosis, hematochezia, hypotension-
related symptoms, and melena or with a positive screening fecal
occult blood test (FOBT) or chronic iron-deficient anemia with
no obvious source of blood loss. Esophagogastroduodenoscopy
(EGD) is the diagnostic examination of choice for upper GI
bleeding and should be performed in most all suspected cases.
Urgency of the initial management is based on the amount and
acuteness of the blood loss. Patients who are hemodynamically
unstable or have active bleeding need to be hospitalized and
managed aggressively, while selected patients who are hemodynamically stable with no evidence of active bleeding may be
managed in an outpatient setting. Upper GI bleeding can be
acute requiring immediate intervention, occult and remain subclinical for years, or obscure which is not readily diagnosed, all
of which may require extensive investigation.

Acute Upper GI Bleeding

The most common cause of acute upper GI bleeding are peptic ulcers, encompassing about 60% of all patients, followed by erosive gastritis (15%), and variceal bleeding (6%). Patients with acute upper GI bleeding usually present with signs of hemodynamic instability, such as dizziness, light-headedness, weakness, pallor, palpitations, tachycardia, orthostatic hypotension, shock, and even cardiopulmonary arrest. Bleeding in these patients is usually evidenced by hematemesis, melena, or even hematochezia which may be found in over 14% of patients with upper GI bleeding.

Initial Assessment

Patients with suspected acute upper GI bleeding should be assessed rapidly and stabilized. Unstable patients and stable patients with active or recent bleeding need a large-bore intravenous (IV) catheter placed during the initial workup. Blood loss needs to be estimated and the bleeding localized. If the patient is unstable, immediate resuscitation should be started.

Resuscitation: The unstable patient with active or recent bleeding needs to be managed aggressively. Airway, breathing, and circulation (the ABCs) should be assessed immediately and appropriate interventions instituted when necessary. Infusion of fluid with 0.9% normal saline or Ringer's lactate (RL) through large-bore IV lines or a central line should be started and blood transfused as needed to maintain tissue perfusion; in elderly patients, the hematocrit should be kept above 30%, while in young, healthy patients, the target hematocrit should be above 20%. A urinary catheter may be needed to monitor urine output, and any coagulopathy should be sought and corrected. These patients should be monitored in an intensive care unit. When the patient stabilizes, an emergent evaluation should be undertaken; however, if the patient remains unstable, the patient should undergo emergent EGD and/or operative intervention, depending on the severity of bleeding and knowledge of the site of bleeding.

Emergent Evaluation

Patient history: Medical history should include investigation of prior episodes of upper gastrointestinal bleeding (ulcers or varices), liver disease, intestinal polyps or cancer, and blood transfusions. Alcohol abuse and illicit drug use should also be investigated. A careful history of medication use must be taken, including use of aspirin, nonsteroidal anti-inflammatory drugs (NSAIDs), and anticoagulation drugs (warfarin, heparin). Symptoms such as abdominal pain, nausea, vomiting, hematemesis, early satiety, anorexia, and weight loss should be sought. A cardiac history is important to determine the threshold for blood transfusion.

Physical examination: Careful attention should be paid to signs of chronic liver disease, such as jaundice, caput medusae, spider telangiectasia, and/or ascites. Physical examination should include a digital rectal examination and an NG tube aspiration. If the NG aspirate is bloody and/or if a non-gastric upper GI source is suspected, an upper GI endoscopy is recommended; if, however, the aspirate is bilious or clear and there is no clinical evidence for upper GI bleeding, a colonoscopy is indicated.

Initial work-up: Initial blood work should include a complete blood count, liver and renal function tests, coagulation parameters (PT/INR, PTT), and typing and crossmatching. Chest and abdominal x-rays are also needed (these tests may indicate perforation or aspiration), and an ECG is warranted, for patients with cardiovascular risk factors. Early risk stratification into high risk or low risk for re-bleeding or mortality using a validated risk scale, such as the Rockall or Baylor risk scales, may be beneficial for the health care team (Table 12.1). If there is a high risk of rebleeding or mortality, the patient should be hospitalized, investigated, and treated. Patients that have a low risk can be managed in an outpatient setting.

TABLE 12.1. Risk factors for upper GI bleeding.

Risk factors for upper GI bleeding
Older age (>60 years)
Severe comorbidity
Active bleeding
Hypotension or shock
Red blood cell transfusion ≥6 units
Inpatient status at time of bleed
Severe coagulopathy
High risk endoscopic stigmata

Emergent Management

Detection and diagnosis: All patients with suspected upper GI bleeding probably require an endoscopy. In the emergent setting, a gentle gastric lavage with warm, 0.9% saline through the NG tube should be performed prior to endoscopy to remove blood and food particulate matter. This irrigation permits better visualization of the upper GI tract and decreases the chance of massive aspiration. EGD not only detects the location of the bleeding but may also diagnose the underlying cause and control the bleeding. If the EGD is negative and an upper GI source is still suspected, a red blood cell-tagged radionucleotide scan should be considered. Barium studies are not indicated in acute upper GI bleeding, because the contrast interferes with endoscopy and potential operation.

Emergent treatment: Variceal bleeding can be treated endoscopically with band-ligation or injection sclerotherapy, which can be used concomitantly with octreotide, somatostatin, or glypressin (octreotide: 50 mg IV bolus followed by 50 mg per 8–24 h; Somatostatin: 250–500 mg IV bolus followed by 250–500 mg per hour; glypressin: 2 mg bolus IV

followed by 1 mg per hour). Endoscopic sclerotherapy combined with this drug therapy is better than sclerotherapy
alone.

Endoscopic hemostasis should always be attempted in
patients with non-variceal bleeding. Hemostasis can be
achieved either by injection sclerotherapy, electrocoagula-
tion, heater probes, or laser therapy. Concomitant drug therapy with high-dose, proton-pump inhibitors (PPI; IV bolus
followed by continuous infusion) improves outcome, decreases
rebleeding rate, and decreases hospital stay. If endoscopic
control fails, radiologic intervention, balloon tamponade, and
operative intervention with or without intra-operative endoscopy should be considered (Fig. 12.1).

Occult Upper GI Bleeding

Upper GI bleeding is not always overt or associated with the
classic signs of hematemesis and melena but may present as
a chronic iron-deficiency anemia or a positive FOBT without any visible bleeding. These patients should stimulate a
high degree of suspicion and should be investigated thoroughly for the source of blood loss. A detailed medical history is fundamental and includes investigation of liver
disease, intestinal polyps or cancer, blood transfusions, alcohol abuse, and illicit drug use. As with acute bleeding, a careful history of medication use including over-the-counter
medication is imperative. Symptoms such as abdominal pain,
nausea, vomiting, early satiety, anorexia, or weight loss
should be sought and careful attention paid to signs of
chronic liver disease.

Colonoscopy and EGD are the first investigations for
occult bleeding; however, in about 50% of patients, the source
of the bleeding is not found. If the EGD shows the underlying
cause, medical, endoscopic, or operative therapy are instituted.
If both colonoscopy and EGD are negative, further immediate investigation may not be necessary especially in younger

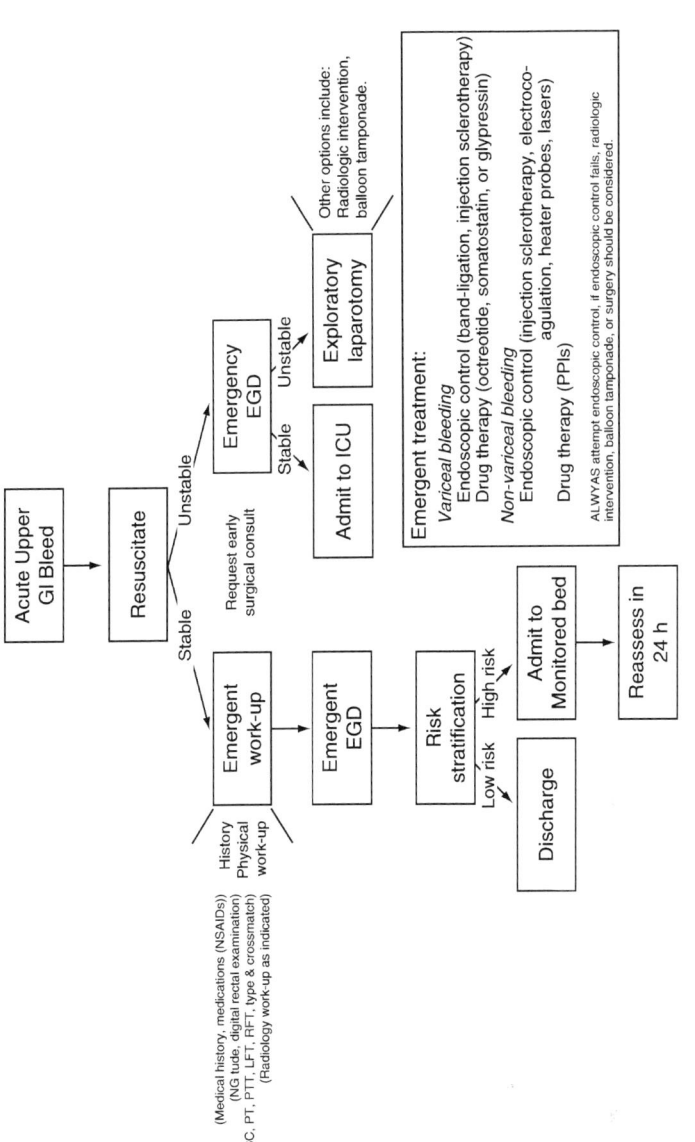

FIGURE 12.1.   Acute upper GI bleeding algorithm.

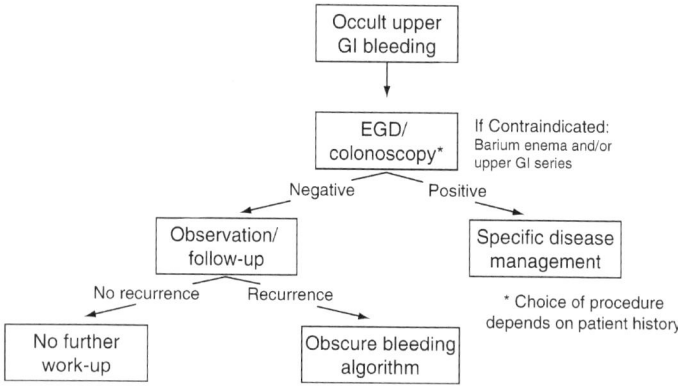

FIGURE 12.2. Occult upper GI bleeding algorithm (Adapted from American Gastroenterological Association medical position statement, 2000. With permission).

patients; however, if positive FOBTs or iron-deficiency persists, further investigation is necessary as described for obscure GI bleeding (Fig. 12.2).

Obscure Upper GI Bleeding

Obscure upper GI bleeding is defined as recurrent overt or occult bleeding after an initial negative endoscopic examination. If the bleeding is overt with evidence of ongoing blood loss, the patient should be evaluated as an acute upper GI bleed; in these patients, a RBC-tagged radionucleotide scan is recommended as part of the diagnostic work-up. For the remaining patients, a repeat endoscopy with enteroscopy is recommended; if negative, these endoscopic modalities should be followed by enteroclysis or small bowel series, and possibly angiography. Finally, if the bleeding persists and diagnostic exams are inconclusive, consideration should be given to exploratory operation with intraoperative enteroscopy.

Diagnostic Modalities

Endoscopy

Conventional EGD: All patients with suspected upper GI bleeding and without any contraindications should eventually undergo an EGD. Gentle gastric lavage with 0.9% normal saline may be needed to remove blood and particulate matter to improve visualization. Erythromycin given intravenously (250 mg IV bolus or 3 mg/kg IV over 20–30 min) 20–90 min before endoscopy improves visibility and decreases endoscopy time. The EGD can detect and diagnose most sources of upper GI bleeding and allows tissue biopsy for pathologic examination and hemostasis. Numerous techniques are available for control of bleeding, including electrocautery, heat probe, laser therapy, band ligation, clip placement, injection sclerotherapy, and injection of cryanoacrylic glue.

Enteroscopy: Visualization of the entire small bowel mucosa remains a challenge to endoscopists. Push enteroscopy, in which an enteroscope is pushed beyond the ligament of Trietz, is the standard approach. This technique has a diagnostic yield of about 60%, because a significant proportion of lesions detected by the enteroscope are within reach of the endoscope. A "second look" EGD may be recommended before an enteroscopy is planned. Newer extended techniques such as double balloon enteroscopy show promising results but remain to be validated. These techniques often do not permit therapeutic intervention and may not provide reliable information of distance from the ligament of Treitz.

Video capsule endoscopy: Video capsule endoscopy is a recent, nearly non-invasive technique in which a small capsule (11 mm with camera, lens, and transmitter) is ingested orally by the patient and transmits images to a receiver. This technique can diagnose a site of bleeding in over 50% of patients with obscure bleeding using negative push endoscopy. Its drawbacks are that it is inefficient in the esophagus and stomach and does not permit tissue sampling, intervention, or clear identification of where exactly in the jejunoileum the abnormality is located. It is, however, an excellent diagnostic tool that should be considered, especially in patients with obscure bleeding in whom an exploratory operation is the next step. On rare occasions, the capsule may become entrapped and require operative removal and therefore should not be used in patients with suspected strictures or known extensive adhesions.

Radiology

Barium contrast series: In the emergency setting, barium studies are contraindicated, because barium interferes with endoscopic and operative visualization. In the elective setting and especially in the investigation of obscure bleeding, a barium contrast series has a high diagnostic yield for small bowel bleeds secondary to a mass lesion and can be used before push enteroscopy in high-risk patients or after a negative push enteroscopy.

Enteroclysis: Enteroclysis is a double-contrast study performed by passing a tube into the proximal small bowel and injecting barium, methylcellulose, and air often in conjunction with intravenous glucagon. This technique has a greater diagnostic yield than conventional imaging because of its increased resolution and lack of an overlapping, barium-filled stomach, but due to patient discomfort, its use is limited. One should consider this technique selectively.

Angiography: Angiography is usually reserved for bleeding that either was not detected by conventional strategies or in patients in whom other treatments have failed. Angiography can detect a bleeding rate of greater than 0.5 ml/min; active bleeding is seen as extravasation of contrast into the lumen of the bowel, but angiography will also show abnormal vessels or vascular blushes even in the absence of active bleeding. Angiography permits selective infusion of a vasoconstrictor, such as vasopressin and/or embolization with gelfoam, polyvinyl alcohol, or a solid blocking material. In hemorrhagic gastritis, selective arterial injection of vasopression should be attempted if medical treatment fails. Angiography with selective intraarterial embolization is the treatment of choice for hemobilia and remains the best method for diagnosis.

Radionucleotide scans: Radionucleotide scans with either Technetium pertechnate-labeled autologous red blood cells or Technetium sulfur colloid can detect bleeding at a rate of 0.1–0.4 ml/min. This technique is extremely sensitive but is less specific than an endoscopy or arteriography and often only localizes the site of bleeding to an area of abdomen. Confirmation with either an arteriography or endoscopy may be necessary.

Operative exploration/intraoperative enteroscopy: Celiotomy for intraoperative endoscopy is the last resort for diagnosing and/or treating acute GI bleeding not detected or amenable to other interventions and for diagnosing thoroughly investigated obscure, recurrent GI bleeding requiring multiple transfusions (Fig. 12.3). Intraoperative enteroscopy is usually best performed by making a mid small bowel enterotomy and examining the bowel lumen proximally and distally during a gradual controlled insertion of the endoscope rather than after telescoping the bowel over the endoscope and examining the mucosa while removing the tube. Passing the endoscope into the small bowel either by mouth or per anus is much less effective and may not allow visualization of the entire jejunoileum.

Management of Specific Causes of Upper GI Bleeding

Peptic Ulcers

Peptic ulcers are the most frequent cause of upper GI bleeding. Aggressive medical therapy with PPIs combined with endoscopic, interventional, therapeutic techniques is extremely effective in controlling the acute phase of peptic ulcer bleeding. The success of this approach may create a dilemma for the surgeon in deciding whether or not to continue with a nonoperative approach or to submit the patient to abdominal

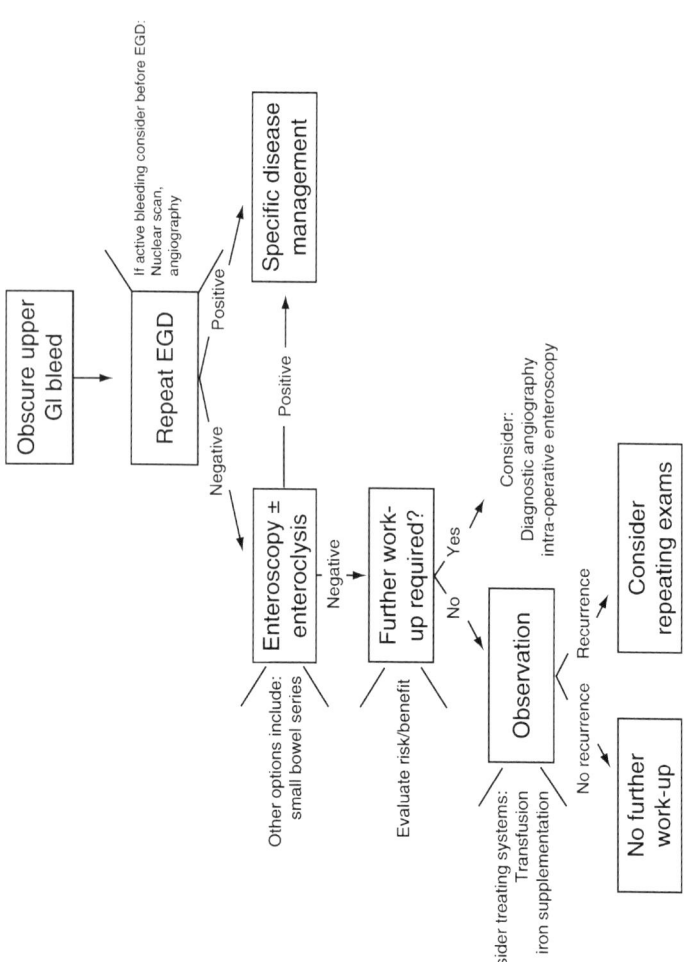

FIGURE 12.3. Obscure upper GI bleeding algorithm (Adapted from American Gastroenterological Association medical position statement, 2000. With permission).

exploration. Endoscopy is the first line therapy; in general, if the patient requires more than 4–6 units of blood and the bleeding is not controlled endoscopically, the patient should be managed operatively. Patients who are hemodynamically unstable and have ongoing hemorrhage should also be treated operatively. Other criteria for operative intervention include a rebleeding ulcer that is not controlled by endoscopy and medical therapy and possibly those patients with giant ulcers and a "visible vessel." All patients with endoscopically confirmed peptic ulcers should be given high-dose, intravenous PPI therapy. Also, if the patient tests positive for H. pylori, antibiotic eradication should be initiated and later confirmed.

Operative intervention can be either laparoscopic or open, depending on the surgeon's expertise, severity of bleed, and the localization of the ulcer. For duodenal ulcers, vessel ligation through a longitudinal duodenotomy over the site of the ulcer is performed. Care must be taken to not injure the common bile duct. In contrast, operative treatment for gastric ulcers includes either hemigastrectomy, usually without vagotomy unless it is a distal antral ulcer, or a wedge resection (usually for proximal lesions) with or without proximal gastric vagotomy considering that long-term PPI therapy may be equivalent to proximal vagotomy.

Mortality and re-bleeding after operative treatment of bleeding peptic ulcers is associated with high rates of mortality and re-bleeding.

For these reasons and due to the efficiency of PPI in treatment of peptic ulcer, more recent trends have been to only suture control the bleeding site and to treat the patient aggressively with, postoperative acid suppression as well as medical treatment of any associated H. pylori infection with the drugs now available.

Variceal Bleeding

Variceal bleeding is responsible for about a third of all cirrhosis-related mortality and must be treated aggressively. Endoscopic hemostasis with band-ligation, injection sclerotherapy, or clip placement is successful in a majority of patients, and the need for emergency porto-systemic shuts has become a treatment of the past. Concomitant drug therapy with octreotide, somatostatin, or glypressin improves bleeding control and outcome(octreotide: 50 mg IV bolus followed by 50 mg per 8–24hrs; Somatostatin: 250–500 mg IV bolus followed by 250–500 mg per hour; Glypressin: 2 mg IV bolus followed by 1mg every 4 hours). If endoscopic control fails, balloon tamponade (Minnesota tube or Sengstaken-Blakemore tube) should be attempted for a maximum 24–48 h followed by endoscopic hemostasis. Once acute bleeding is controlled, treatment with propranolol (40 mg, p.o., b.i.d.) should be initiated; sclerotherapy or band ligation of remaining varices should be performed at weekly intervals until all varices are sclerosed or ligated.

Operative therapy should be avoided whenever possible in patients who are candidates for liver transplantation. If bleeding persists in these patients, a transjugular intrahepatic portosystemic shunt (TIPS) to decompress the portal system is often preferable. This procedure, however, is associated with a mortality of about 10% and hepatic encephalopathy around 20%; therefore, its application is recommended as a bridge to liver transplantation. If bleeding persists or recurs and medical and endoscopic measures fail, then operative intervention is required, but this scenario has become quite uncommon. Patients who are not candidates for liver transplantation and who are stable should undergo a distal splenorenal shunt if the venous anatomy is appropriate; if not, a mesocaval graft, a porto-caval shunt, or a gastric devascularization with esophageal transection is recommended.

Patients with Schistosomiasis

In patients with portal hypertension secondary to mansonic schistosomiasis, endoscopic sclerosis or rubber banding of bleeding esophageal varices achieve good results in over 90% of patients. Should recurrent bleeding occur, then the operative strategy is to interrupt the left gastric vein and to devascularize the greater curvature of the stomach, and to perform a splenectomy followed by endoscopic sclerosis of esophageal varices.

If varices of the gastric wall are present, it is necessary to oversew the varicose veins through a gastrotomy; treating these specific lesions with endoscopy alone has limited success. Recurrence of bleeding after transgastric ligation of bleeding gastric varices at follow-up of 30 months was 15% and overall mortality was 6%. In portal hypertension due to liver cirrhosis, the approach of azygous-portal disconnection is not considered an adequate procedure, because it is followed by a very high rate of re-bleeding as well as high risk of portal thrombosis.

Hemorrhagic Gastritis

Severe bleeding from gastritis has become extremely rare. Most bleeding from gastritis is almost always controlled medically with PPIs, H_2 receptor blockers, antacids, and/or sucralfate. If medical treatment fails, administration of vasopressin via the left or right gastric arteries should be attempted. In this setting, if medical therapy fails, the results of operative intervention are quite poor, and every attempt should be made to avoid need for operative intervention. If severe bleeding persists, a total or sub-total gastrectomy may be required, however, the need for such an aggressive approach has virtually disappeared. It is for this reason that prophylaxis against stress gastritis for ICU patients with either PPIs or an H2 receptor blocker is recommended. All patients with gastritis should undergo H. pylori screening, and if positive, treatment should be initiated; follow up confirmation of eradication of *H. pylori* is highly recommended.

Mallory-Weiss Tears

Mallory-Weiss tears result from repeated vomiting. In most patients, the bleeding stops without therapy. If bleeding persists, endoscopic coagulation may be necessary. Only rarely is operative intervention required for direct suture of the tear which can be done through a high anterior gastrotomy.

Neoplasms

Clinically important, acute bleeding due to neoplasms of the upper GI tract is not common. Some patients with gastric cancer, particularly in early stages, may develop gastric bleeding followed by hematemesis, particularly in patients taking NSAIDs or aspirin. The endoscopic examination should be used to biopsy the lesion to confirm the diagnosis. Usually the bleeding stops spontaneously. Hemorrhage due to advanced gastric cancer that erodes the left gastric artery or another vascular pedicle of the stomach, although rare, may be severe and persistent, making an operative intervention mandatory to resect the tumor or at least to obliterate the bleeding vessel if the malignancy is non-resectable.

Acute bleeding due to an esophageal neoplasm is very rare, although in some instances, advanced carcinoma of the lower third of the esophagus can erode the descending aorta provoking a catastrophic, but terminal hemorrhage.

Gastrointestinal stromal tumors (GIST) may provoke acute bleeding as the first symptom of the disease. The bleeding is usually self-limited, giving time for the diagnosis of site and origin of the blood loss. The treatment is almost always operative, even if palliative, but newer chemotherapeutic options have become available, offering prolonged effective palliation in some of these patients.

Lymphoma is another important cause of bleeding in the GI tract; however, hemorrhage from these lesions usually is not continuous, making the diagnosis and the staging of the disease possible followed by the establishment of a treatment strategy, which is often multidisciplinary.

Adenomas of the upper GI tract, more often located in the small bowel (especially periampullary) but occurring also in the stomach and rarely in the esophagus, may be caused of intense GI bleeding. Treatment may be endoscopic resection or operative.

Hiatus Hernia and Esophagitis

Esophagitis and hiatus hernia are very rare causes of acute upper GI bleeding as opposed to chronic bleeding; their diagnosis is easily made by endoscopy. Treatment in the acute phase is usually the same as for non-complicated esophagitis and achieves good results in general terms.

Vascular Lesions

Dieulafoy lesions: Dieulafoy's lesion typically presents with intermittent, recurrent, acute upper GI bleeding. The lesion occurs when an abnormally large-caliber submucosal artery becomes exposed at the surface of the mucosa and then ruptures, usually in the stomach, but on occasion in the small bowel. Diagnosis may be quite difficult, even in the stomach, because the lesion is focal and bleeds only intermittently. In contrast, preoperative diagnosis from a lesion in the small bowel requires either endoscopic visualization or demonstration by angiography. Endoscopic methods to treat Dieulafoy's lesion include banding, clipping, electrocautery, cyanoacrylate glue injection, sclerosant injection, epinephrine injection, heat probe, banding, and laser therapy. Angiographic embolization can be tried as well. If these therapies fail, operative control is indicated.

Aortoenteric fistulas: Most aortoenteric fistulas occur secondary to erosion into the bowel from a pseudoaneurysm that has formed from the proximal aortic anastomosis after prior placement of an intraabdominal aortic graft; primary aorto-enteric fistulas, although exceedingly rare, can occur from an atherosclerotic or mycotic aortic aneurysm. Most aortoenteric fistulas occur at the level of the distal duodenum or the jejunum and sometimes the colon. These lesions require operative intervention.

Vascular ectases: Vascular ectasias or angiodysplasia may be cause of acute GI bleeding but are much more common in the large bowel in older patients. In contrast, small bowel vascular lesions are usually arteriovenous malformations and occur in younger patients <40 years old. When in the stomach or upper part of the duodenum, the hemorrhagic episode may be treated by endoscopic methods. Recently with the development of therapeutic enteroscopes, some patients with bleeding of small bowel arteriovenous malformations have been treated successfully.

Hemobilia

Loss of blood through biliary tree directly into the duodenal lumen is a very rare condition. Hemobilia is usually secondary to operative trauma, prior percutaneous biliary intubation. The diagnosis is usually made by angiography and treated by arterial embolization. Liver neoplasms may also cause hemobilia.

Selected Readings

Adler DG, Leighton JA, Davila RE et al. (2004) ASGE guideline: The role of endoscopy in acute non-variceal upper-GI hemorrhage. Gastrointest Endosc 60:497–504

American Gastroenterological Association medical position statement (2000) Evaluation and management of occult and obscure gastrointestinal bleeding. Gastroenterology 118:197–201

Barkun A, Bardou M, Marshall JK (2003) Consensus recommendations for managing patients with nonvariceal upper gastrointestinal bleeding. Ann Intern Med 139:843–857

British Society of Gastroenterology Endoscopy Committee (2002) Non-variceal upper gastrointestinal haemorrhage: guidelines. Gut 51(Suppl 4):iv1–6

Esrailian E, Gralnek IM (2005) Nonvariceal upper gastrointestinal bleeding: epidemiology and diagnosis. Gastroenterol Clin North Am 34:589–605

Ferguson CB, Mitchell RM (2005) Nonvariceal upper gastrointestinal bleeding: standard and new treatment. Gastroenterol Clin North Am 34:607–621

Ferraz AAB, Lopes EPA, Barros FMR et al. (2001) Splenectomy þ left gastric vein ligature þ devascularization of the great curvature of the stomach in the treatment of hepatosplenic schistosomiasis. Postoperative endoscopic sclerosis is necessary? Arq Gastroenterol 38:84–88

Legrand MJ, Jacquet N (1996) Surgical approach in severe bleeding peptic ulcer. Acta Gastroenterol Belg 59:240–244

Manning-Dimmitt LL, Dimmitt SG, Wilson GR (2005) Diagnosis of gastrointestinal bleeding in adults. Am Fam Physician 71:1339–1346

Rockey DC (2005) Occult gastrointestinal bleeding. Gastroenterol Clin North Am 34:699–718

Sava G, Marescaux J, Grevier JF (1980) Place de la vagotomie tronculaire avec hémostase local dans le traitement de l'ulcere duodénale hémorragique. J Chir (Paris) 117:683–687

Triadafilopoulos G (2005) Review article: the role of anti-secretory therapy in the management of non-variceal upper gastrointestinal bleeding. Aliment Pharmacol Ther 22(Suppl 3):53–58

Part IV
Minimally Invasive Procedures

13
Laparoscopic Appendectomy

Jason F. Hall and Richard Hodin

Pearls and Pitfalls

- Laparoscopic appendectomy can be safely performed in most patients, even in the setting of perforated appendicitis.
- Laparoscopic appendectomy generally takes slightly longer than the conventional, open approach, although with experience, there is little or no difference in operative time.
- Benefits of laparoscopic appendectomy include a decreased incidence of wound infection, possibly a shorter hospital stay, and better exposure in the obese patient.
- Interval appendectomy is accomplished easily using the laparoscopic approach.
- In the case of an appendiceal mass, either open appendectomy or initial medical management are most appropriate.
- Surgeons performing laparoscopic appendectomy should be familiar with endoscopic stapling and suturing techniques.
- Complications of laparoscopic appendectomy are similar to those of the open procedure and can be managed in the same fashion.
- Many surgeons, once familiarized with laparoscopic appendectomy, maintain that the visualization is far superior than with open appendectomy.

K.I. Bland et al. (eds.), *Surgery of the Small Bowel*,
DOI: 10.1007/978-1-84996-372-5_13,
© Springer-Verlag London Limited 2011

Open appendectomy has been the standard of care for the management of acute appendicitis since its description by McBurney in 1894. Semm first described laparoscopic appendectomy in 1981, and since that time, the technique has endured debate related to its cost, efficacy, and safety. Although a multitude of non-randomized and randomized trials have compared the two procedures, no clear consensus has emerged in the surgical community regarding the superiority of either technique. Taken together, however, the results of the various trials suggest that laparoscopic appendectomy has some advantages over the open procedure. Patients undergoing laparoscopic appendectomy appear to have lower rates of wound infection, less post-operative pain, and a shorter duration of stay. Laparoscopic appendectomy is, however, generally associated with a longer operative time and higher hospital costs/charges (Table 13.1). Many authors have argued that a small incision in the right lower quadrant is already minimally invasive and also has the advantage of being easy to perform without the need for fancy laparoscopic equipment. In contrast, experienced surgeons find the

TABLE 13.1. Results from meta-analyses of prospective randomized trials comparing laparoscopic and open appendectomies (Reprinted from Chung RS, et al, 1999. Copyright 1999. With permission from Elsevier).

	Operative time (min)	Hospital days	Recovery days	Wound infection	Post-operative abscess
Number of trials analyzed	17	17	12	15	15
Laparoscopic appendectomy	63	3.1	11.4	3%	2%
Open appendectomy	48	3.5	17	7%	1%
Significant difference (p < 0.001)	Yes	No	Yes	Yes	No

laparoscopic approach to be quick and easy (similar to the experience with laparoscopic cholecystectomy), especially when performed frequently in an individual hospital, such that operating room personnel become familiar with the equipment and setup. Moreover, the concept of a "minimally invasive" approach appeals to the public and can be a very effective marketing strategy.

Indications for Operation

The indications to perform a laparoscopic appendectomy are essentially the same as those for the open procedure. A complete history and physical examination are required. Periumbilical abdominal pain, followed by anorexia/nausea/vomiting, which then progresses to localized tenderness at McBurney's point in the right lower quadrant, represents the classic and most common presentation, occurring in approximately 50 percent of patients with acute appendicitis. Many patients display specific findings on physical examination, including Rovsing's sign (localized right lower quadrant pain on palpation of the left lower quadrant) and/or Dunphy's sign (pain with coughing or movement). When perforation occurs, these symptoms progress to generalized peritonitis, although some patients will "wall off" the process and present with a localized phlegmon or abscess. A pelvic and retrocecal appendix often produces atypical symptoms associated with an obturator or psoas sign. Patients with appendicitis usually have fever and leukocytosis, although these may be absent in the early stages. It is our practice to always check a urine pregnancy test in females of child bearing age. Although laparoscopic appendectomy is not contraindicated in pregnancy, knowledge of this condition may influence the method of entry into the abdomen (Hassan trocar vs. Veress needle) and the presence of pneumoperitoneum attained.

While the history and physical examination are sufficient to make the diagnosis of appendicitis, abdominal computed tomography (CT) has become an integral part of the evaluation of the majority of these patients in many centers. Although CT is highly sensitive and specific (up to 100% and 97%, respectively) for the detection of acute appendicitis, the negative appendectomy rate has not decreased from the pre-CT era. Abdominal CT does, however, have the ability to image an alternative intra-abdominal diagnosis. Although the majority of patients at many institutions are evaluated with abdominal CT before operation for appendicitis, a normal CT scan does not entirely exclude the diagnosis, especially early in the course of inflammation. The common findings of appendicitis include a dilated appendix (>6 mm in diameter), peri-appendiceal inflammation and stranding, cecal wall thickening, and if intravenous contrast is used, appendiceal wall enhancement. CT can also help predict possible failure of laparoscopic appendectomy, because severe inflammation on CT (grade 4 or 5, i.e., an appendix with surrounding fat stranding or an inflammatory mass or abscess) may suggest a 20% chance of conversion to open appendectomy (Table 13.2).

Once the diagnosis of acute appendicitis is established, urgent removal of the appendix is the treatment of choice in the Western world, although in many countries in Asia, non-operative treatment with intravenous antibiotics may be preferred. In patients with an established abscess or phlegmon, especially when the history suggests that the process has been present for more than 3–5 days, non-operative management with antibiotics and possible CT-guided drainage is an excellent approach. Such patients would then be candidates for possible interval appendectomy at a later time.

TABLE 13.2. Predictors of conversion from laparoscopic to open appendectomy (Reprinted from Liu S, et al., 2002. Copyright 2002. With permission from Elsevier).

Predictor	Odds ratio	95% CI	p
Age ≥ 65 years	3.9	1.2–12.5	0.023
Diffuse tenderness	8.4	1.1–67	0.045
Surgeons with 10 LA	4.1	1.3–13.0	0.016
CT grade	2.8	1.2–6.2	0.013

Outcome Measures in Laparoscopic Appendectomy

In the past few years, many prospective randomized trials and meta-analyses comparing laparoscopic and open appendectomy have been published. In general, the results indicate that laparoscopic appendectomy is associated with a shorter hospital stay. Several large trials have demonstrated earlier return to work (3 and 6 days) after laparoscopic appendectomy, but discharge to home and return to work are measures that can be influenced by many factors, including the expectations of the patient and/or medical team.

Many studies show that patients undergoing laparoscopic appendectomy are less likely to have a post-operative wound infection (OR 0.45; CI95% 0.35–0.58). Most studies show no increase in intra-abdominal abscess formation after laparoscopic appendectomy.

The duration of operation has generally been longer with a laparoscopic approach (approximately 12 min), and costs are also greater. Several groups, however, have pointed out that there are reduced societal costs with the laparoscopic approach because of earlier return to work.

Equipment

Laparoscopic appendectomy is usually performed using a 30°, 5 or 10 mm laparoscope, one 5 mm trocar, and one 12 mm trocar. A sharp dissector, atraumatic bowel forceps, electrocautery, and a laparoscopic stapler are necessary. We use the vascular 2.0 mm staples for the mesoappendix and the 3.0 mm staples for the appendix itself. A laparoscopic clipping device, looped suture, and specimen retrieval bag can be used as well.

Positioning and Preparation

The patient is positioned supine. Some surgeons prefer to tuck the left arm at the patient's side. The bladder should be decompressed, either by having the patient void prior to the procedure or by placing a bladder catheter. Lateral rather than midline placement of trocars in the lower abdomen will avoid bladder injury. If the diagnosis is unclear in a young woman, the lithotomy position may be preferable to allow for better visualization of the uterus and ovaries. DVT prophylaxis with subcutaneous heparin and/or pneumoboots should be employed. Broad-spectrum antibiotics are given within 2 h of the start of the procedure.

Trocar Placement

In general, only three trocars are necessary. We prefer the technique of open pneumoperitoneum via a periumbilical incision to minimize any chance of bowel or vascular injury. The 12 mm port is then placed under laparoscopic vision in the left lower quadrant and a 5 mm port in the right lower quadrant (Fig. 13.1). Alternatively, one can use a 5 mm port in the left lower quadrant and then use that port for a 5 mm

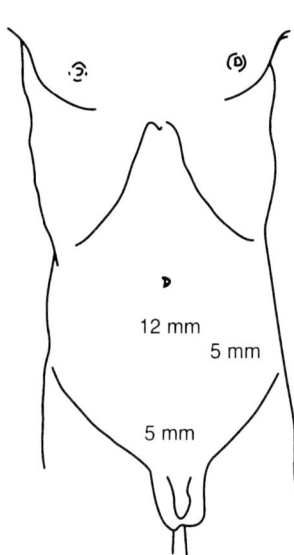

FIGURE 13.1. Placement of the operative ports for laparoscopic appendectomy is shown. A 5 or 10/12 mm port can be used inter-changeably in the infraumbilical or suprapubic positions.

laparoscope and the larger periumbilical port for the stapler. Other trocar placements have been described, but the general principle is to allow triangulation of the working instruments on the appendix without obstructing the camera.

Operative Procedure

Once the pneumoperitoneum is established, the peritoneal cavity is inspected. The patient is placed in Trendelenburg position with the left side down. If the appendix is retrocecal, the white line of Toldt should be taken down using electrocautery. Injury to the ureter and retroperitoneal vessels are avoided by staying close to the cecal wall during this dissection. Once identified, the appendix is traced back to its origin on the cecum. There is usually a small avascular window between the mesoappendix and the base of the appendix that can be opened with the sharp dissector, and the vascular 2 mm stapler can be used to divide the mesoappendix. In some circumstances, it is easier to control the appendix itself prior to the mesoappendix. When firing the endoscopic staplers, one must ensure that no extra structures are included in the jaws of the stapler. The mesoappendix can also be divided retrograde starting at the tip of the appendix. This technique, in general, requires use of the vascular load for the stapler. Occasionally, the mesoappendix and the appendix are extraordinarily inflamed and are difficult to manipulate. Under these circumstances, a looped suture or an endoloop can be introduced via a 14 gauge catheter in the right lower quadrant and placed around the tip of the appendix to allow for manipulation. Once the mesoappendix is divided, the base of the appendix is dissected, and any filmy adhesions are divided with a cautery. Once the base is cleared, the appendix can be divided with a 3.0 mm tissue stapler. One must be careful to dissect down to the true base of the appendix, because incomplete excision of the appendix can lead to "stump appendicitis" within the remaining appendix. The staple line must be placed in healthy cecal wall. If severe inflammation is present, the stump should be inverted using intra-corporeal suturing,

or the procedure should be converted to an open appendectomy. The staple line should be inspected for leaks or bleeding. Electrocautery should be used minimally if at all on the
staple line, so as to avoid damage to the cecal wall.

Once the appendix and mesoappendix have been divided,
the appendix should be removed from the abdomen either in
a specially designed laparoscopic bag or into the detached
index finger of a sterile surgical glove externalized through
the 12 mm port. Alternatively, the appendix can be pulled
into the lumen of the 12 mm trocar and removed by pulling
the entire appendix/port complex out of the abdomen. We
close all port sites greater than 10 mm with 0 polyglactin
suture and with subcuticular sutures.

Thorough irrigation of the right lower quadrant should be
performed in all patients. In cases of perforation, one should
attempt to irrigate clean the peritoneal cavity to the extent
possible. It is likely that laparoscopy provides better visualization of the pelvis and the remaining peritoneal cavity compared to the McBurney incision, allowing for a more complete
irrigation of the sepsis. Drains are almost never used.

If on exploratory laparoscopy the appendix is normal, and
there are no other identifiable causes of abdominal pain, we
still remove the appendix. If there is another explanation
found, such as endometriosis, diverticulitis, or a perforated
ulcer, the normal appendix should probably be left alone.

Postoperative Care

Patients who had bladder catheters placed pre-operatively
typically have them removed before leaving the operating
room. The patient can be started safely on a liquid diet and
advanced to a regular diet within 24 h. Assuming that the
patient is tolerating regular food, requiring minimal narcotics,
and able to ambulate, they can be discharged within 24 h. In
gangrenous or perforated appendicitis, we administer a few
days of oral antibiotics. In simple appendicitis, however, no
additional antibiotics are administered after operation.

Complications

The complications of laparoscopic appendectomy are the same as those associated with the open procedure. In addition, the procedure carries those risks associated specifically with laparoscopy.

Complications described after laparoscopic appendectomy include wound infection, intra-abdominal abscess, ureteral injury, vascular injury, enteric injury, and deep vein thrombosis.

Special Situations in Laparoscopic Appendectomy

Elderly patients: Laparoscopic appendectomy applied strictly to elderly populations has not been well studied. Recent publications suggest that laparoscopic appendectomy is well tolerated by elderly patients and maintains several of the advantages identified in other groups. Specifically, elderly patients who underwent laparoscopic appendectomy had a shorter duration of stay, higher rate of routine discharge, lower complication rate, and lower mortality in comparison to patient who had the open procedure.

Pregnancy: The published experience with laparoscopic appendectomy in pregnancy is not extensive and is limited to small series and case reports. A review of the literature would suggest that the procedure is well tolerated by the mother and fetus. One recent review identified 94 cases in the literature. There was one fetal death associated with the laparoscopic approach, and the complication rate was lower than that typically associated with the open procedure. Initial trocar placement should be performed using an open (Hassan) technique to avoid the gravid uterus, and intra-abdominal pressures should not exceed 14 mmHg. Pregnant patients should be managed in conjunction with the obstetrical service with fetal monitoring pre-, intra-, and post-operatively.

Interval laparoscopic appendectomy: Patients managed initially with non-operative treatment of a periappendiceal abscess traditionally will undergo an interval appendectomy. Interval laparoscopic appendectomy can be performed safely and easily. If sufficient time has elapsed since the initial disease process (at least 8–10 weeks), generally little or no periappendiceal inflammation will be found. Patients can be discharged usually on the same day as the procedure.

Obese patients: Although obesity was once considered a contraindication to laparoscopic appendectomy, surgeons have gained more experience with the technique, and the data now suggest that these patients recover more quickly compared with the open procedure. Obesity should not be considered a contraindication to laparoscopic appendectomy, and indeed, may be an indication for a laparoscopic approach.

Appendiceal masses: Appendiceal neoplasms are rare, but surgeons must have a clear approach for resecting them if they are encountered during operation. Evidence suggests that carcinoid neoplasms can be resected safely with a laparoscopic technique. Patients with small neoplasms (<2 cm) located away from the appendiceal base can be treated laparoscopically. In contrast, if a larger mass is evident or there is concern about the margins of resection, conversion to an open procedure would be appropriate if the surgeon is not comfortable with a laparoscopic ileo ascending colectomy.

Selected Readings

Balthazar EJ et al. (1991) Appendicitis: prospective evaluation with high-resolution CT. Radiology 180:21–24

Chung RS et al. (1999) A meta-analysis of randomized controlled trials of laparoscopic versus conventional appendectomy. Am J Surg 177:250–256

Enochsson L (2001) Laparoscopic vs. open appendectomy in overweight patients. Surg Endosc 15:387

Hellberg A et al. (1999) Prospective randomized multicenter trial of laparoscopic versus open appendectomy. Br J Surg 86:48

Liu S et al. (2002) Factors associated with conversion to laparotomy in patients undergoing laparoscopic appendectomy. J Am Coll Surgeons 194:298–305

Mun S et al. (2006) Rapid CT diagnosis of acute appendicitis with IV contrast material. Emerg Radiol 12:99–102

Pedersen AG et al. (2001) Randomised controlled trial of laparoscopic versus open appendectomy. Br J Surg 88:200

Sauerland S et al. (2006) Laparoscopic versus open surgery for suspected appendicitis. The Cochrane Collaboration (Review)

Silen W (1996) Cope's early diagnosis of the acute abdomen, 19th edn. Oxford University Press, New York

14
Laparoscopic Small Bowel Surgery

Elisabeth C. McLemore and Tonia M. Young-Fadok

Pearls and Pitfalls

- The root of the small bowel mesentery lies directly beneath the umbilicus, facilitating exteriorization of the small bowel via a small periumbilical incision.
- Use of gravity and repositioning of the operating table facilitate inspection of the entire small bowel.
- In the emergent setting, small-bowel obstruction may be approached laparoscopically in selected patients without tense abdominal distension.
- Small-bowel resection and side-to-side stapled anastomosis can be performed using only two firings of a linear stapler.
- Enterotomies made using sharp dissection frequently bleed and/or leak and are recognizable at the time of operation. Enterotomies caused by electrical or ultrasonic energy may go unrecognized at the time of operation as they are sealed temporarily, and may not leak under the pressure of the pneumoperitoneum.
- Gastrointestinal (GI) bleeding identified by angiography can be localized with injection of methylene blue through the catheter for specific intraoperative localization.

K.I. Bland et al. (eds.), *Surgery of the Small Bowel*,
DOI: 10.1007/978-1-84996-372-5_14,
© Springer-Verlag London Limited 2011

Small Bowel Anatomy and Pathology

Anatomy

Two features of small bowel anatomy create challenges for laparoscopic approaches. The combination of the length of the small intestine (6–15 ft) and the ladder-like arrangement of multiple loops of the small bowel means that the entire small bowel cannot be visualized with the limited view provided by the laparoscope. Thus, evaluation of the entire length of the small bowel requires careful technique to remain oriented and not become confused regarding which loop has already been examined.

One feature of the anatomy of the small intestine does serve to facilitate laparoscopic procedures. Because the root of the small bowel mesentery lies directly beneath the umbilicus, almost any loop of small intestine can be exteriorized through a small (3–5 cm) periumbilical incision. Once the cecum and terminal ileum have been mobilized, such an incision allows for exteriorization of the small intestine almost in its entirety to a point approximately 3–5 cm distal to the ligament of Treitz.

Pathology

The diagnosis of small bowel pathology is often elusive because imaging requires a size and mass threshold for diagnosis, and endoscopic evaluation is limited. The most common indication for operative intervention on the small intestine is obstruction from adhesions. Obstruction may be caused less commonly by incarcerated small bowel within a hernia, Crohn's disease, foreign body, intussusception, radiation stricturing, or metastatic deposits from other intra-abdominal malignancies, or from primary neoplasms such as melanoma and breast cancer. The majority of small bowel neoplasms are malignant (60–70%) and include carcinoid neoplasms, lymphomas, adenocarcinoma, and GI stromal neoplasms. Benign neoplasms of the small bowel include adenomas, lipomas, and hemangiomas. Less common pathology includes duplication cysts, malrotation, Meckel's diverticulum, and small bowel polyps in Peutz-Jeghers syndrome. The small bowel is the most frequently injured hollow viscus in both blunt and penetrating abdominal trauma.

Operative Indications and Contraindications

The decision for either a laparoscopic or open approach to small bowel disease is dependent on the indication and the surgeon's level of experience. The indications for laparoscopic procedures of the small intestine are identical to open procedures. The most common indication for operative intervention for small bowel pathology is obstruction secondary to adhesions. In the acute setting, tense abdominal distension often precludes the ability to establish a pneumoperitoneum. This provides functional working space intraperitoneally. In the situation where some degree of decompression has been obtained with nasogastric suction, a laparoscopic approach can be considered.

Crohn's disease, while initially considered to be too complex for laparoscopic approaches, has been found to be well suited to minimally invasive techniques, particularly in the setting of limited ileocecal disease. The presence of complex disease, with associated fistula, abscess, or phlegmon, does not preclude a laparoscopic approach, but will increase the risk of conversion to an open procedure.

Malignant neoplasms of the small intestine are rare and should be approached with caution and maintaining correct oncologic technique. Use of the laparoscopic approach for small bowel adenocarcinomas distal to the ligament of Treitz retains an element of controversy as a consequence of lessons learned from wound implants seen early in the history of laparoscopic resection for colon adenocarcinoma. However, as the pathology is frequently not established preoperatively, excellent oncologic techniques with appropriate margins,

extent of lymphadenectomy, and avoidance of tumor handling are important. Small bowel lymphomas, carcinoid neoplasms, and GI stromal neoplasms do not have a propensity
toward abdominal wall recurrence, and laparoscopic resection is an option.

Laparoscopy in upper GI bleeding should only be considered if the source of bleeding has been identified. Bleeding
from a Meckel's diverticulum may be confirmed by a technetium pertechnetate scan. GI bleeding identified by angiography can be localized intraoperatively if the angiography
catheter has been left in place after subselective catheteriza-
tion; after anesthetization and establishment of pneumoperitoneum, methylene blue can be injected intra-arterially via
the catheter to identify the segment of interest.

Hemodynamic instability and coagulopathy are considered
absolute contraindications to laparoscopic intervention by
most authors. Extensive fecal and purulent peritonitis may not
be adequately managed laparoscopically due to difficulties irri-
gating all loculated fluid collections adequately. Laparoscopy
during pregnancy in the second trimester is generally considered safe, but long-term clinical studies are lacking, and laparoscopy during pregnancy should be approached with caution.

Preoperative Patient Preparation

After a thorough history and physical examination in the
elective setting, workup proceeds as for an open procedure to
ensure that the patient is in optimal condition for an operation. A full evaluation of the upper and lower GI tract is
performed in patients with Crohn's disease. If malignancy is
suspected, a metastatic workup should be performed. If there
is a history of prior abdominal surgery, a review of the operative notes may be helpful in discovering if extensive adhesions were present previously.

Although a bowel preparation may not be performed
prior to an open approach, a preparation is often preferred
prior to a laparoscopic approach so that minimal residual
fluid remains in the small intestine, allowing the small bowel

loops to be handled more easily. In the emergent setting, with small-bowel obstruction, a bowel preparation is contraindicated. Intravenous antibiotics are given within 60 min prior to the incision and discontinued within 24 h postoperatively.

Operative Techniques

Instrumentation

Standard laparoscopic equipment includes a laparoscope angled at 30°, energy source, and appropriate instruments for handling of the bowel. The surgeon's familiarity with the energy source utilized determines safety more so than the type of energy source used. When instruments are well maintained and insulating casings are checked for defects, the authors have found the use of monopolar scissors with minimal use of electrocautery for adhesiolysis and the dissection of soft tissue planes to be without complications, faster, and cheaper than other energy sources. Enterotomies made using sharp dissection bleed and/or leak frequently and are recognizable at the time of surgery. Enterotomies made using electrical or ultrasonic energy sources may go unrecognized at the time of operation as these enterotomies are temporarily sealed.

Gentle handling of the bowel is more important than the type of bowel grasper used, especially with the thin-walled bowel during a bowel obstruction. Even atraumatic instruments may create serosal tears or enterotomies in careless hands. Grasping the adjacent peritoneum rather than the bowel itself and using the grasper as a retractor are other techniques that minimize bowel injury. With these techniques, inadvertent enterotomies can be avoided, and two simple 5 mm Babcock or atraumatic graspers suffice in most situations.

Abdominal Entry and Exploration

The patient is placed in the supine position. Orogastric or nasogastric and bladder decompression are used in almost all patients. Multiple techniques for abdominal access have been described, including cut-down techniques distant from prior incisions (our preference), use of a viewing trocar, and creation of the pneumoperitoneum via closed insertion of a Veress needle in the left subcostal position. In the patient without prior abdominal surgeries, we have found that the supraumbilical cut-down technique is simple, reliable, and can be incorporated into a periumbilical incision for bowel excision/exteriorization when necessary.

Exploration and small bowel resection are commenced with three ports triangulated toward the right lower quadrant: a 12 mm camera port in the supraumbilical midline, and two 5 mm ports in the left lower quadrant and the suprapubic midline (Fig. 14.1). An additional port in the right lower quadrant can be placed as necessary. Two monitors are utilized, one placed on each side of the operating table.

Applications

Small Bowel Evaluation

There are two methods for laparoscopic evaluation of the small bowel. The first method, intracorporeal instrument evaluation, is of limited thoroughness. Intracorporeal evaluation is acceptable for inspection of the bowel for serosal tears or enterotomies following lysis of adhesions and for localization of obvious pathology, such as a Meckel's diverticulum. The technique may miss more subtle findings such as the web-like strictures sometimes seen with treated Crohn's disease or with nonsteroidal antiinflammatory drugs. Because the ileocecal valve is identified readily with the patient in left-side-down and Trendelenburg position, it is often easiest to begin evaluation of the small intestine at this point and proceed proximally to the ligament of Treitz in a retrograde fashion. Using two bowel graspers, a hand-over-hand instrument technique can be performed passing each successive segment of bowel from one clamp to the other. If both instruments are kept within the field of vision, a dropped segment of

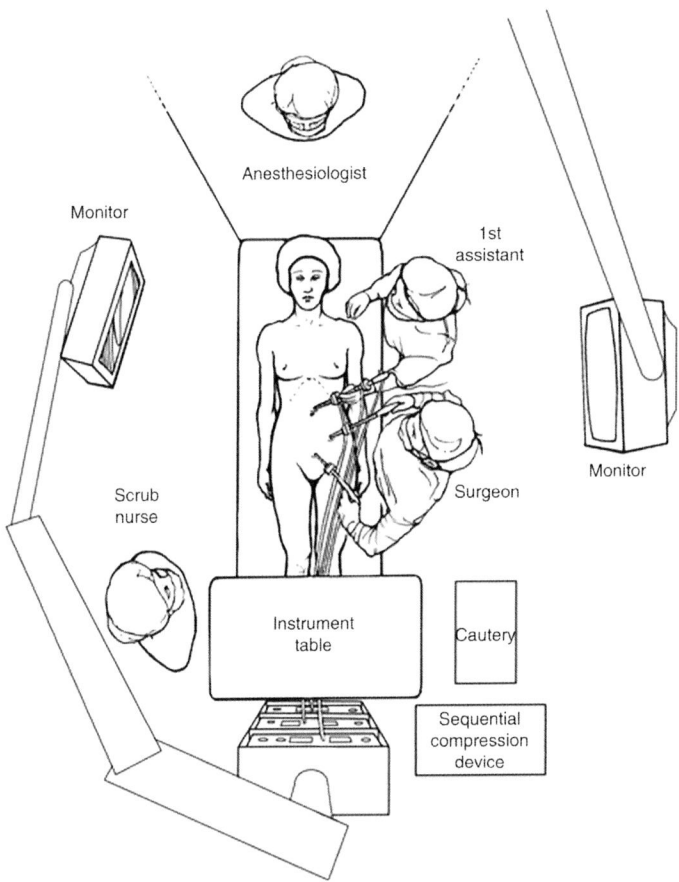

FIGURE 14.1. Trocar placement and operating room set up. Three ports triangulated toward the right lower quadrant are placed: a 12 mm camera port in the supraumbilical midline and two 5 mm ports in the left lower quadrant and the suprapubic midline. After trocar placement, the surgeon and first assistant stand on the patient's left side.

bowel can be easily retrieved and the hand-over-hand technique continued. This approach will limit the need to start the evaluation all over again due to uncertainty regarding which loop of bowel was previously in the grasper. Moreover, traumatic injuries to the bowel are better recognized if both graspers remain in view at all times. As the mid small bowel is reached, a more neutral position followed by right-side-down and reverse Trendelenburg position will facilitate examination of the proximal small bowel and identification of the ligament of Treitz. Orienting one of the monitors on the left at the head of the bed instead of at the foot of the bed aids this part of the examination.

The second method for evaluation of the small bowel is exteriorization of the small bowel through a small 3–5 cm periumbilical incision for extracorporeal evaluation and palpation. This approach is our preferred method in any setting in which a small-bowel resection is performed or a more thorough evaluation of the small intestine is indicated, as in Crohn's disease. The cecum must be mobilized to allow the ileocecal valve to be exteriorized. The entire small bowel up to a point approximately 4–5 cm from the ligament of Treitz can be evaluated extracorporeally; this incision also allows for deployment of a long tube with inflatable balloon (e.g., Baker tube) to detect strictures.

Small Bowel Obstruction

A similar port placement is used for exploratory laparoscopy for small bowel obstruction. In the presence of a midline incision, the supraumbilical midline is involved frequently by adhesions. Our preference is to place the initial port using a cut-down technique in either upper quadrant and subsequent ports are placed under direct vision. Extensive or dense adhesions may preclude a laparoscopic approach. Laparoscopic treatment of acute adhesive small bowel obstruction should be approached with caution. The rate of conversion to an open approach is high, approximately 45–52%, either because intestinal distension obscures the field of vision or adhesions are too extensive. The reported risk of small bowel perforation is increased in the laparoscopic approach.

Adhesions are lysed carefully from the anterior abdominal wall. The 30° laparoscope, facing upward, facilitates visualization of adhesions. Gentle counter traction of the adhesions with one instrument and sharp dissection without cautery of adhesions with the other hand facilitates identification of the correct plane of dissection. Soft sweeping motions also facilitate identification of the proper plane. In some instances, extracorporeal application of focal point external pressure on the abdominal wall may assist in bringing adhesions into a more easily accessible position.

When faced with extensive or dense adhesions, a guideline for conversion to open is helpful. Suggestions include conversion to open if there is a lack of timely progress, inability to identify anatomy safely, and the surgeon's own sense of growing frustration.

Small Bowel Resection

Small bowel resection is begun typically with three ports triangulated toward the right lower quadrant as described above. After initial exploration, the patient is placed in the left-side-down Trendelenburg position, which helps the small bowel and omentum to fall into the left upper quadrant away from the operative field. To perform ileocecectomy, as opposed to a limited small bowel resection, the cecum must be mobilized. Mobilization of the ascending colon facilitates exteriorization and allows for a wide, side-to-side stapled anastomosis. The correct retroperitoneal plane is entered by scoring the peritoneum around the base of the terminal ileal mesentery and the cecum. The right lateral peritoneal reflection is opened, and the ascending colon is mobilized medially. The entire small bowel can be exteriorized through a periumbilical extraction incision in most patients. To facilitate exteriorization in obese patients and to perform an oncologic resection in patients in whom malignancy is suspected, the mesentery should be divided intracorporeally.

After the small bowel is exteriorized and the mesentery has been divided, the resection and side-to-side stapled anastomosis can be performed with two firings of an 80 or 100 mm linear stapler. The proximal and distal sites of resection are placed side to side. An enterotomy is made at the antimesenteric end of both proximal and distal sites of resection. The first firing of the stapler is used to create the new side-to-side anastomosis. After hemostasis has been confirmed, the second firing of the stapler is used to resect the small bowel specimen and simultaneously close the side-to-side anastomosis (Fig. 14.2). The side-to-side anastomotic configuration overlies the mesenteric defect, which is not closed. The small bowel is returned to the abdominal cavity. The trocar sites are inspected for hemostasis by reestablishing a pneumoperitoneum and removing the trocar sites under direct laparoscopic vision or by elevating the periumbilical incision and using the laparoscopic light to provide illumination.

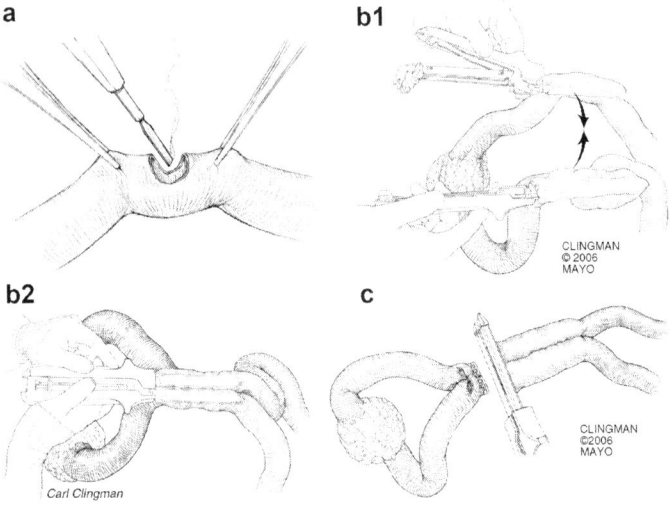

FIGURE 14.2. Two application technique of linear stapler for a side-to-side anastomosis. (**a**) An enterotomy is made on the antimesenteric end of both proximal and distal sites of resection. (**b1** and **b2**) The first firing of the linear stapler creates the side-to-side anastomosis. (**c**) The second firing of the stapler is used to resect the small bowel specimen and simultaneously close the side-to-side anastomosis.

Totally intracorporeal laparoscopic small bowel resections have been described. An extraction incision is still required to remove the specimen, however, and there are no recognized advantages of this technique over exteriorization of the small bowel for specimen resection. In fact, this technique is more expensive, because it uses more staple firings and more trocars, and is associated with increased operative time and increased risk of spillage of intraluminal contents compared with the exteriorization method. The segment of bowel to be resected is grasped between two bowel clamps and elevated to display the mesentery. The mesentery is scored and individual vessels are ligated with clips, staples, or bipolar or ultrasonic scissors. The bowel is transected with an endoscopic stapler and placed into a protective bag for immediate or delayed retrieval via a port site that has been enlarged minimally for extraction. An intracorporeal side-to-side stapled anastomosis is performed by aligning the two transected ends of bowel along their antimesenteric boarder. A small enterotomy is made in the antimesenteric end of each staple line, and a 60 mm laparoscopic linear stapler is insinuated carefully into the lumen of each intestinal limb. The remaining confluent defect can be closed with the use of a laparoscopic stapler or intracorporeal sutures.

Ileocolic Resection for Crohn's Disease

As noted above, mobilization of the cecum and ascending colon facilitates exteriorization and allows creation of a wide side-to-side stapled anastomosis. Resection of the typically thickened Crohn's mesentery is often more safely performed extracorporeally. The small bowel can be exteriorized in its entirety after the cecum and ascending colon are mobilized and evaluated for more proximal areas of disease. Significant weblike strictures may be present with minimal extraluminal findings, such as serosal injection, bowel wall thickening, or creeping fat. These strictures can be missed by intracorporeal evaluation. Exteriorization of the small bowel and deployment of a Baker tube (a long tube with an inflatable balloon at the end) at a planned point of resection or strictureplasty will often allow discovery of these significant strictures. The same principles apply to laparoscopic-assisted strictureplasty with full evaluation of the entire small intestine extracorporeally, facilitated by mobilization of the cecum. A Baker tube is utilized to identify all areas of stricturing in diffuse disease. Extracorporeal strictureplasty is performed readily.

Meckel's Diverticulum

Meckel's diverticulectomy is indicated for bleeding, inflammation, palpable mass, or obstruction. In adults, the most common presentation is obstruction from intussusception, volvulus, or inflammatory adhesions. The extent of small bowel resection for Meckel's diverticulum is determined by the associated disease process. A laparoscopic-assisted diverticulectomy can be performed with two ports: one camera port and one working port to identify and grasp the diverticulum. The diverticulum is elevated with the grasper and exteriorized through a very small periumbilical extraction incision for extracorporeal resection. A segmental resection of the diverticulum can also be performed using this technique. Alternatively, total intracorporeal diverticulectomy can be performed with three ports. The diverticulum is identified and elevated, the vascular supply clipped or cauterized depending on the vessel size, and a laparoscopic stapler fired across the base. The stapler should be fired in a direction transverse to the longitudinal axis of the bowel lumen to prevent compromise of the luminal diameter.

Small Bowel Ischemia

Exploratory laparoscopy is a valuable tool for evaluation of suspected small bowel ischemia. Laparoscopic evaluation allows for confirmation of the diagnosis and evaluation of the extent of small bowel infarction. The decision to proceed with small bowel resection versus a palliative approach can often be made with one or two port placements. In addition, second-look laparoscopy can be performed in the intensive care setting if the ports left in situ for subsequent access are maintained under sterile conditions.

Small Bowel Intussusceptions

Intussusceptions in adults should be considered secondary to a malignant neoplasm serving as the lead point until proven otherwise. Laparoscopic reduction of the intussuscepted intestine should probably not be performed in adults, especially if there is worry about viability of the intussuscepted segment, because this reduction may cause inadvertent enterotomy or tumor spillage. Therefore, mobilization of the terminal ileum and cecum to allow exteriorization of the intussuscepted small bowel via a 3–4 cm periumbilical incision is performed using proper oncologic technique to prevent abdominal wall recurrence. The intussuscepted small bowel is then assessed for lead point root cause, and an appropriate resection can be performed extracorporeally.

Small Bowel Foreign Body

Bezoars, a conglomeration of food or foreign material in the alimentary tract, or gallstones are the most common type of GI foreign bodies. The incidence of small-bowel obstruction from intraluminal foreign bodies is less than 5%. Adults with previous gastric procedures, incomplete mastication, delayed gastric emptying or stasis, hypothyroidism, intestinal diverticulum, adhesive bands, and stricture may be predisposed to bezoar formation. Similarly, gallstone ileus can be suspected in older patients with small bowel obstruction who have no history of hernia or previous abdominal surgery; pneumobilia may be a clue to this diagnosis. Exploration and small bowel evaluation can be performed with three ports triangulated towards the right lower quadrant as described above. Once the transition point has been identified, the offending bezoar is located, gentle extramural fragmentation of the bezoar is performed using atraumatic graspers or forceps, and the fragmented bezoar is transported to the cecum. Unlike bezoars, gallstones require enterotomy and removal, but the remainder of the small bowel should be examined carefully for other gallstones. Usually the cholecystoduodenal fistula is not dealt with acutely. All of these steps can be performed extracorporeally via a small periumbilical incision if there is suspicion of intraluminal pathology, if the bezoar cannot be fragmented, or if there is evidence of small bowel perforation.

Evaluation of Small Bowel Injury in Blunt Abdominal Trauma

Hollow viscus injury after blunt abdominal trauma is uncommon. The relative risk of small bowel injury is more than doubled in patients with the so-called seat-belt sign and/or flexion-distraction fractures of the spine (Chance fractures). The use of CT and selective laparoscopy in the diagnosis and management of bowel injury in blunt abdominal trauma is gaining interest as a means of preventing a nontherapeutic laparotomy and avoiding delayed diagnosis in patients with suspected blunt bowel injury.

Diverting Loop Ileostomy

Temporary fecal diversion can be achieved with a diverting loop ileostomy. While blindly creating an ileostomy site and utilizing the closest loop of small bowel has been described in the literature (trephine approach), this approach risks complications, because the ileostomy may be twisted inadvertently, it may be difficult to identify the most distal loop of the small bowel, and adhesions may prevent this approach. A two-port laparoscopic approach minimizes the risk of these potential complications. The stoma site is marked preoperatively in the right lower quadrant by a stoma therapist.

A disk of skin and fat is excised at the marked stoma site, the anterior rectus sheath is opened in a cruciate fashion, and the longitudinal muscle fibers are separated. A purse-string suture is placed around the posterior rectus sheath entry site and used to secure a blunt port. A pneumoperitoneum is established, and a 5 mm port is placed in the left lower quadrant under direct vision. The 5 mm camera is then switched to the left lower quadrant port. With the patient in a left-side-down Trendelenburg position the terminal ileum is identified, and using a bowel grasper or clamp via the right lower quadrant port, an appropriate loop of small bowel can be brought up through the stoma site under direct vision. This approach ensures that the loop is oriented correctly and free of tension. The ileostomy is matured in standard fashion.

Postoperative Management

The orogastric tube is removed in the operating room. Perioperative antibiotic prophylaxis is discontinued within 24 h postoperatively. Postoperative pain control is initiated with intravenous analgesic agents. Deep vein thrombosis (DVT) prophylaxis is continued perioperatively in the form of compressive stockings, sequential compression devices, and early ambulation. Subcutaneous administration of unfractionated heparin or low-molecular weight heparin for DVT prophylaxis is utilized as appropriate.

After lysis of adhesions, loop ileostomy, or Meckel's diverticulectomy, clear liquids can be resumed the day of the operation and advanced as tolerated to a regular diet and oral analgesia the following day. The patient is ready for discharge usually on the first or second postoperative day.

After a small bowel resection, ileocolic resection, or stricturoplasty, clear liquids can often be initiated on the first postoperative day if the patient is not nauseated or exhibiting abdominal distension. A regular diet is resumed the following day and postoperative pain control can be converted to an oral analgesic agent. The patient is ready for discharge on postoperative day two or three.

Surgical Outcomes

In general, laparoscopic techniques are associated with decreased postoperative pain, decreased duration of hospital stay, and earlier return to activities of daily living. Postoperative pain appears to be less as indicated by reduced analgesic requirements compared to conventional laparotomy. Postoperative ileus after small bowel resection is frequently of shorter duration after a laparoscopic approach. The shorter duration of postoperative ileus may be due to decreased narcotic use, reduced handling of the small bowel, and limited exposure to evaporative losses and the cooler ambient temperature of the operating room. The rate of surgical site infection has also decreased with the laparoscopic approach. While the long-term results are equivalent at this point, there is a decreased propensity for adhesion formation with the laparoscopic approach, and the incidence of postoperative bowel obstruction may be reduced.

After laparoscopic lysis of adhesions, the average duration of stay is 2.5 days. The rate of conversion to an open operation is around 25%, most frequently prompted by extensive adhesions. Missed enterotomy continues to be the most feared complication. Persistent postoperative fever or leukocytosis, prolonged ileus, or peritoneal signs should prompt a thorough evaluation for missed enterotomy.

Laparoscopic exploration and lysis of adhesions in patients with chronic abdominal pain and no documented episodes of small bowel obstruction is extremely controversial. In 2003, Swank and colleagues reported their results from a blinded, randomized, controlled multicenter trial of 100 patients randomized after laparoscopy to adhesiolysis versus no further intervention. Both groups reported a substantial relief in pain and improved quality of life. The authors concluded that diagnostic laparoscopy alone was of the same benefit to laparoscopic adhesiolysis in the relief of chronic abdominal pain.

Laparoscopic techniques have become widely accepted for Crohn's disease, and particularly for limited ileocolic disease. In a randomized controlled trial of laparoscopic-assisted or open ileocolic resection for Crohn's disease, there was no difference between the two groups in the primary outcome parameter, postoperative quality of life measured by SF-36 and GIQLI questionnaires, during 3 months of follow up; however, secondary endpoints such as morbidity, duration of stay, and costs were significantly lower. We have noted similar outcomes.

Selected Readings

Maartense S, Dunker MS, Slors JF et al. (2006) Laparoscopic assisted versus open ileocolic resection for Crohn's disease: a randomized trial. Ann Surg 243:143-149; discussion 150–153

Mitsuhide K, Junichi S, Atsushi N et al. (2005) Computed tomographic scanning and selective laparoscopy in the diagnosis of blunt bowel injury: a prospective study. Journal of Trauma-Injury Infection & Critical Care 58:696-701; discussion 701–703

Rivas H, Cacchione RN, Allen JW (2003) Laparoscopic management of Meckel's diverticulum in adults. Surg Endosc 17:620–622

SAGES Committee on Standards of Practice (2000) SAGES guidelines for laparoscopic surgery during pregnancy. SAGES Publication #0023, 2000, http://www.sages.org/sagespublication.php?doc=23

Swank DJ, Swank-Bordewijk SC, Hop WC et al. (2003) Laparoscopic adhesiolysis in patients with chronic abdominal pain: a blinded randomised controlled multi-centre trial. Lancet 361:1247–1251

Wullstein C, Gross E (2003) Laparoscopic compared with conventional treatment of acute adhesive small bowel obstruction. Brit J Surg 90:1147–1151

Yau KK, Siu WT, Law BK et al. (2005) Laparoscopic approach compared with conventional open approach for bezoar-induced small-bowel obstruction. Arch Surg 140:972–975

Young-Fadok TM, HallLong K, McConnell EJ et al. (2001) Advantages of laparoscopic resection for ileocolic Crohn's disease. Improved outcomes and reduced costs. Surg Endosc 15:450–454

Index